Ophthalmologica

International Journal of Ophthalmology
Journal International d'Ophtalmologie
Internationale Zeitschrift für Augenheilkunde

Organ of the Netherlands Ophthalmological Society

Founded 1899 as 'Zeitschrift für Augenheilkunde'
by H. Kuhnt and J. von Michel
Continued by J. Meller (1923–1938), C. Behr (1925–1938),
A. Brückner (1938–1959), H.J.M. Weve (1938–1962),
H.M. Dekking (1954–1966), J. ten Doesschate (1967–1971),
J. François (1959–1979), E.B. Streiff (1954–1979), H. Sautter (1979–1984)

Publication data: 'Ophthalmologica' is published 8 times annually. Volumes 198–199 with 4 issues each appear in 1989.
Subscription rates: Subscriptions run for a full calendar year. Prices are given per volume, surface postage included.
Personal subscription: SFr. 163.10, US$ 105.00. (Must be in the name of, billed to, and paid by an individual. Order must be marked 'personal subscription'.)
Institutional subscription: SFr. 233.–, US$ 150.00. (Regular rate.)
Members of the Schweizerische Ophthalmologische Gesellschaft; Netherlands Ophthalmological Society: SFr. 139.80, US$ 90.00.
Airmail postage: SFr. 25.–, US$ 18.00. (Extra per volume.)
Microform subscription: SFr. 116.50, US$ 75.00. (Available exclusively to subscribers of the paper edition.)
Single issues and back volumes: Information on availability and prices can be obtained through the Publisher.

Subscription orders: Orders can be placed at agencies, bookstores, directly with the Publisher S. Karger AG, P.O. Box, CH – 4009 Basel (Switzerland) or with any of the following distributors:
Deutschland, West-Berlin, Ost-Europa, Naher Osten: S. Karger GmbH, Postfach 1724, D – 8034 Germering/München
France: Librairie Luginbühl, 36, bd de Latour-Maubourg, F – 75007 Paris
Great Britain: John Wiley and Sons, Ltd., Baffins Lane, Chichester, Sussex, PO19 1UD
USA: S. Karger Publishers, Inc., 79 Fifth Avenue, New York, NY 10003
India, Bangladesh, Sri Lanka: S. Karger India Subscription Agency, B – 5/132 Safdarjung Enclave, New Delhi-110029
Japan, South Korea: Katakura Libri, Inc., 36-9 Hongo 3-chome, Bunkyo-ku, Tokyo 113
Change of address: Both old and new address should be stated and sent to the subscription source.

Bibliographic indices: This journal is regularly listed in bibliographic services, including *Current Contents®*.
Book Reviews: Books are accepted for review by special agreement.
Advertising: Correspondence and rate requests should be addressed to the Publisher.

KARGER

Ophthalmologica
Printed in Switzerland

S. Karger AG,
Postfach, CH – 4009 Basel (Schweiz)

Erscheint anderthalbmonatlich;
pro Jahr 2 Bände zu 4 Heften

Ophthalmologica

Submission: Only original papers written in English, French or German are considered and should be sent to:

Prof. Dr. Dr. W. Straub
Universitäts-Augenklinik
Robert-Koch-Strasse 4
D-3550 Marburg a.d. Lahn (FRG)

Manuscripts should be submitted in duplicate (with two sets of illustrations of which one is an original), typewritten double-spaced on one side of the paper, with a wide margin.

Conditions: All manuscripts are subject to editorial review. Manuscripts are received with the explicit understanding that they are not under simultaneous consideration by any other publication. Submission of an article for publication implies the transfer of the copyright from the author to the publisher upon acceptance. Accepted papers become the permanent property of 'Ophthalmologica' and may not be reproduced by any means, in whole or in part, without the written consent of the publisher. It is the author's responsibility to obtain permission to reproduce illustrations, tables, etc. from other publications.

Arrangement:

Title page: The first page of each paper should indicate the title (main title underlined), the authors' names, and the institute where the work was conducted. A short title for use as running head is also required.

Key words: For indexing purposes, a list of 3-10 key words in English is essential.

Abstract: Each paper needs an abstract in English of up to 10 lines.

Summary: Papers written in either French or German must be accompanied by a summary in the same language of not more than 10 lines.

Small type: Paragraphs which can or must be set in smaller type (case histories, test methods, etc.) should be indicated with a 'p' (petit) in the margin on the left-hand side.

Footnotes: Avoid footnotes. When essential, they are numbered consecutively and typed at the foot of the appropriate page.

Tables and illustrations: Tables and illustrations (both numbered in Arabic numerals) should be prepared on separate sheets. Tables require a heading and figures a legend, also prepared on a separate sheet. For the reproduction of illustrations, only good drawings and original photographs can be accepted; negatives or photocopies cannot be used. When possible, group several illustrations on one block for reproduction (max. size 140 × 188 mm) or provide crop marks. On the back of each illustration, indicate its number, the author's name, and 'top'. Color illustrations are reproduced at the author's expense.

References: In the text identify references by Arabic numerals [in square brackets]. Material submitted for publication but not yet accepted should be noted as 'unpublished data' and not be included in the reference list. The list of references should include only those publications which are cited in the text. Do not alphabetize; number references in the order in which they are first mentioned in the text. The surnames of the authors followed by initials should be given. There should be no punctuation other than a comma to separate the authors. When there are more than 3 authors, the names of the first 3 only are used, followed by 'et al'. Abbreviate journal names according to the Index Medicus system. (Also see International Committee of Medical Journal Editors: Uniform requirements for manuscripts submitted to biomedical journals. Ann Intern Med 1982;96: 766-771.)

Examples

(a) Papers published in periodicals: Kauffman HF, van der Heide S, Beaumont F, et al: Class-specific antibody determination against *Aspergillus fumigatus* by means of the enzyme-linked immunosorbent assay. III. Comparative study: IgG, IgA, IgM ELISA titers, precipitating antibodies and IgE binding after fractionation of the antigen. Int Arch Allergy Appl Immunol 1986;80:300-306.

(b) Monographs: Matthews DE, Farewell VT: Using and Understanding Medical Statistics. Basel, Karger, 1985.

(c) Edited books: Hardy WD Jr, Essex M: FeLV-induced feline acquired immune deficiency syndrome: A model for human AIDS; in Klein E (ed): Acquired Immunodeficiency Syndrome. Prog Allergy. Basel, Karger, 1986, vol 37, pp 353-376.

Full address: The exact postal address complete with postal code of the senior author must be given. If correspondence is handled by someone else, indicate this accordingly.

Further details: Authors may consult our leaflet 'Rules for the Preparation of Manuscripts', available on request from the Publisher, S. Karger AG, P.O. Box, CH-4009 Basel (Switzerland).

Page charges: A charge of SFr. 115.- / US $ 75.00 per page will be levied for the first 6 printed pages of an article. Each additional complete or partial page is charged to the author at SFr. 225.- / US $ 150.00. The allotted size of a paper is equal to approx. 12 manuscript pages (including tables, illustrations and references).

Galley proofs: Unless indicated otherwise, galley proofs are sent to the first-named author and should be returned to the publisher with the least possible delay. Alterations made in galley proofs, other than the correction of printer's errors, are charged to the author. No page proofs are supplied.

Reprints: Order forms and a price list are sent with the galley proofs. Orders submitted after the issue is printed are subject to considerably higher prices. Allow five weeks from date of publication for delivery of reprints.

KARGER

Developments in Ophthalmology (ISSN 0250–3751), **Vol. 16**
Series Editor: W. Straub, Marburg a.d. Lahn

Proliferative Vitreoretinopathy/ Genetics of Glaucoma

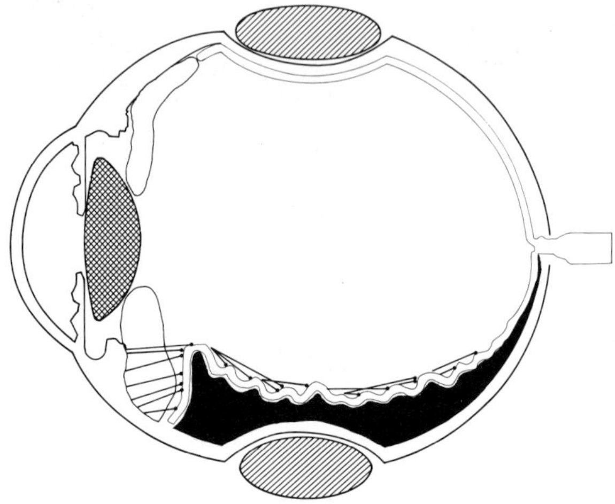

Editor: W. Straub,
Marburg a.d. Lahn

This volume contains three extensive reports on recent advances in the study of proliferative vitreoretinopathy (PVR) together with far-reaching data on the genetics of primary congenital glaucoma. The first chapter examines the pathogenesis of PVR toward identifying those factors which mediate the initiation, development and termination of the events which lead to PVR, knowledge which is critical to the design of therapeutic agents to prevent or ameliorate the disease. The second chapter presents recent findings in immunochemical studies of periretinal membranes, and discusses future applications of immunochemistry leading to improved understanding of the natural course of retinal membrane formation. Chapter three reports the results of studies into the epidemiology and genetics of primary congenital glaucoma (PCG). The investigation tests the hypothesis that PCG in Gypsies is a separate, homogenous form of the disease, and elucidates to what extent heterogeneity can be assumed in the rest of the population.
Bringing together new findings and review data by recognized authorities, these thoroughly referenced articles provide reliable information for all those interested in PVR disorders and in the epidemiology and genetics of congenital glaucoma.

Contents

Fields of Interest

Ophthalmology; Epidemiology, Genetics

Developments in Ophthalmology, Vol. 16
Proliferative Vitreoretinopathy/Genetics of Glaucoma
Editor: Straub, W. (Marburg a.d. Lahn)
approx. VIII + 120 p., 37 fig., 3 cpl., 14 tab., hard cover, 1989
SFr. 114.– / DM 137.– / US$ 76.00
US$ price for USA only (subject to change)
ISBN 3-8055-4853-2

KARGER

KI 89515

Hypertensive Retinopathy

Guest Editor:
Sohan Singh Hayreh, Iowa City, Iowa

35 figures, 7 tables, 1989

KARGER

S. Karger · Medical and Scientific Publishers
Basel · München · Paris · London · NewYork · New Delhi · Singapore · Tokyo · Sydney

Drug Dosage

The authors and the publisher have exerted every effort to ensure that drug selection and dosage set forth in this text are in accord with current recommendations and practice at the time of publication. However, in view of ongoing research, changes in government regulations, and the constant flow of information relating to drug therapy and drug reactions, the reader is urged to check the package insert for each drug for any change in indications and dosage and for added warnings and precautions. This is particularly important when the recommended agent is a new and/or infrequently employed drug.

Printed in Switzerland by
Buchdruckerei Friedrich Reinhardt AG, Basel
ISBN 3-8055-4996-2

Contents

Ophthalmologica 1989;198:173–177

0030–3755/89/1984–0173 $ 2.75/0

Hypertensive Retinopathy

Introduction

Sohan Singh Hayreh

Department of Ophthalmology, University of Iowa Hospitals and Clinics, Iowa City, Iowa, USA

Since Liebreich [1], in 1859, first described 'albuminuric retinitis' in malignant arterial hypertension, hypertensive fundus changes have been regarded as an important part of the syndrome of malignant arterial hypertension. These changes have been given different names. Volhard and Fahr [2], in 1914, called them 'angiospastic retinopathy', a term also advocated later on by Wagener and Keith [3]. Fishberg and Oppenheimer [4], in 1930, called it 'hypertensive neuroretinopathy', which was later abbreviated to 'hypertensive retinopathy'. Wagener et al. [5], in 1947, suggested that different terminologies should be used for various types of hypertensive retinopathy, and these included retinopathy of: acute hypertension/chronic hypertension/terminal malignant hypertension. Finally, 'hypertensive retinopathy' came to be regarded as a universal term for all the fundus changes seen in any type of arterial hypertension. However, our studies [6–11] revealed that from the pathogenetic point of view, the various fundus lesions in malignant arterial hypertension consist of three distinct categories; (1) hypertensive retinopathy, (2) hypertensive choroidopathy, and (3) hypertensive optic neuropathy. Thus, optic disk edema, which was regarded as a very important sign of hypertensive retinopathy, in fact represents hypertensive optic neuropathy and is not a part of hypertensive retinopathy [10]. Similarly, the various retinal pigment epithelial lesions (e.g., the so-called Elschnig's spots), serous retinal detachment and some instances of macular edema represent manifestations of hypertensive choroidopathy [11].

A colossal amount of literature has accumulated on hypertensive retinopathy since its first description in 1859 [1]. In 1871, Allbutt [12] gave an admirable description of it and reviewed the already impressive collection of literature on the ophthalmoscopic and histopathologic findings of almost all the lesions seen in this condition. It is beyond the scope of this introduction to present even a bird's-eye view of the literature. Suffice it to say that, in spite of innumerable publications, hypertensive retinopathy is still the focus of many controversies. Our ability to produce experimentally malignant hypertension and hypertensive retinopathy in primates [8], the advent of fluorescein fundus angiography and its application in hypertensive retinopathy [13–19], and other modern investigative techniques have helped greatly to improve our understanding of this condition. In the papers published in this issue of *Ophthalmologica,* we describe and discuss, in the light of our studies, many of the lesions of hypertensive retinopathy seen in malignant arterial hypertension *(but not in benign arterial hypertension)* and their pathogenesis, as well as some of the major controversies [20–24].

The retinal lesions which constitute hypertensive retinopathy, for descriptive purposes, can be divided into the following vascular and extravascular retinal lesions, although in some of the latter the primary factor may be retinal vascular derangements:

A: *Retinal vascular lesions*
1. Focal intraretinal periarteriolar transudates [9]
2. Cotton-wool spots (inner retinal ischemic spots) [21]
3. Retinal arteriolar changes [20]
4. Retinal capillary changes [21]
5. Retinal venous changes [25]
6. Increased permeability of the retinal vascular bed

B. *Extra vascular retinal lesions*
1. Retinal and macular edema [22]
2. Retinal hemorrhages [25]
3. Retinal lipid deposits ('hard exudates') [23]
4. Retinal nerve fiber loss [21]

For a full understanding of the pathogeneses of the various retinal lesions in hypertensive retinopathy associated with malignant arterial hypertension, one has to bear in mind some of the basic anatomical and physiological properties of the retina and retinal vessels. The properties include the following:

Retinal Arterioles. In the retina the so-called 'retinal arteries' are in fact arterioles, because they possess the following anatomic properties, typically seen in arterioles: (1) the widest part of the lumen of the retinal arterioles is near the optic disk and there its diameter is about 100 μm [26], which is typically the diameter of an arteriole; (2) unlike arteries, they possess neither an internal elastic lamina nor a continuous muscular coat [26, 27].

Absent Autonomic Nerve Supply. It is generally agreed that the vessels in the retina have no adrenergic vasomotor nerve supply [28–30]. However, in a recent study [31], blood vessels lying on the inner surface of the retina in rabbits were claimed to have sympathetic innervation originating from the superior cervical ganglion, distributed in the arterioles from the optic disk to the periphery and also in a few veins; these nerve fibers were numerous near the optic disk and sparse on the peripheral vessels. In view of the overwhelming evidence against the existence of such innervation in man and primates, and also the possibility of species difference, further confirmation of these latest findings is required.

Presence of Autoregulation. The object of autoregulation in a tissue is to keep the blood flow relatively constant during changes in its perfusion pressure. A number of studies have shown the presence of autoregulation in the retina [32–37]. The exact mechanism responsible for the autoregulation is still obscure but it is considered to be a feature of arterioles, particularly the terminal arterioles. With the rise or fall of blood pressure (BP) beyond the normal levels, the arterioles constrict or dilate, respectively, to regulate the blood flow. However, autoregulation becomes ineffective when the BP rises or falls beyond certain limits. With chronic malignant hypertension, the autoregulation adjusts itself to higher than normal levels as a compensatory mechanism, so that the breakthrough of autoregulation may occur at comparatively higher BP levels than in normal persons [38, 39]; we discussed the importance of this at length elsewhere [10].

Presence of Blood-Retinal Barrier. This is well established and is produced by the tight junctions between the endothelial cells of the retinal vessels (duc to the presence of extensive zonulae occludentes) [40, 41]. The tight interendothelial cell junctions block movement of macromolecules from the lumen toward the interstitial space. With a severe rise of BP (i.e. above the level of autoregulation), the autoregulation breaks down, resulting in focal or generalized dilatation of arterioles [9]. Morphological studies of the dilated segments have revealed endothelial cell loss, discontinuity of the endothelial cell layer or interendothelial separation as the initial event. These changes result in the failure of the blood-retinal barrier and increased permeability. The subject of breakdown in the blood-retinal barrier in malignant arterial hypertension is discussed at length elsewhere [9]. Tight cell junctions between the retinal pigment epithelial cells also produce a blood-retinal barrier, preventing the leakage of fluid from the choroid into the retina; this barrier breaks down when the eye develops hypertensive choroidopathy [11]; the role of breakdown of the blood-retinal barrier in the retinal pigment epithelium in the production of the various retinal lesions is also discussed at length elsewhere [11, 22, 23]. The retinal tissue itself has no barrier in its stroma so that fluid may be able to diffuse from one part to the adjacent parts.

Blood Column of Retinal Vessels. As elsewhere in the blood vessels in the body, in the retinal blood vessels the blood flow is fastest in the axial part of the blood column, while it is almost stationary in the peripheral shell, which is in contact with the vessel wall. Also the cells in the blood concentrate in the axial stream, the peripheral part of the blood column being mainly plasma. Ophthalmoscopy or color photographs of the retinal vessels show only the width of the central column of red blood cells. On the other hand, fluorescein fundus angiography reveals the entire width of the blood column, including the peripheral column of plasma.

Relevance of Experimental Studies on Hypertensive Retinopathy in Primates to Man. Finally, the inevitable question arises about the relevance of our experimental studies on hypertensive retinopathy in renovascular malignant arterial hypertension in primates (reported by us in the various papers in this issue) to man. There are no apparent differences between the human and primate in this area of their systemic and ocular anatomy, physiology or other relevant factors, including those discussed above; it would therefore seem logical to conclude that the findings of our experimental studies in primates are equally valid for man. This is further suggested by the close similarities between the hypertensive fundus lesions which we have observed in patients with malignant arterial hypertension, and in our experimental animals. In the experimental studies we were able to do systematic, detailed studies which are not usually possible in man and thus our experimental studies provide information which we may be missing in man.

References

1 Liebreich R: Ophthalmoskopischer Befund bei Morbus Brightii. Graefes Arch Clin Exp Ophthalmol 1859;5:265–268.

2 Volhard F, Fahr KT: Die Brightsche Nierenkrankheit: Klinik, Pathologie und Atlas, vol 8 Berlin, Springer, 1914.

3 Wagener HP, Keith NM: Diffuse arteriolar disease with hypertension and the associated retinal lesions. Medicine (Baltimore) 1939;18:317–430.

4 Fishberg AM, Oppenheimer BS: The differentiation and significance of certain ophthalmoscopic pictures in hypertensive diseases. Arch Intern Med 1930;46:901–920.

5 Wagener HP, Clay GE, Gipner JF: Classification of retinal lesions in the presence of vascular hypertension. Trans Am Ophthalmol Soc 1947;45:57–73.

6 Kishi S, Tso MOM, Hayreh SS: Fundus lesions in malignant hypertension. I. A pathologic study of

experimental hypertensive choroidopathy. Arch Ophthalmol 1985;103:1189–1197.
7 Kishi S, Tso MOM, Hayreh SS: Fundus lesions in malignant hypertension. II. A pathologic study of experimental hypertensive optic neuropathy. Arch Ophthalmol 1985;103:1198–1206.
8 Hayreh SS, Servais GE, Virdi PS, et al: Fundus lesions in malignant hypertension. III. Arterial blood pressure, biochemical and fundus changes. Ophthalmology 1986;93:45–59.
9 Hayreh SS, Servais GE, Virdi PS: Fundus lesions in malignant hypertension. IV. Focal intra-retinal periarteriolar transudates. Ophthalmology 1986;93: 60–73.
10 Hayreh SS, Servais GE, Virdi PS: Fundus lesions in malignant hypertension. V. Hypertensive optic neuropathy. Ophthalmology 1986;93:74–87.
11 Hayreh SS, Servais GE, Virdi PS: Fundus lesions in malignant hypertension. VI. Hypertensive choroidopathy. Ophthalmology 1986;93:1383–1400.
12 Allbutt TC: On the Use of the Ophthalmoscope in Disease of the Nervous System and of the Kidneys; Also in Certain Other General Disorders. London, Macmillan, 1871;213–237.
13 Dollery CT, Hodge JV, Engel M: Studies of the retinal circulation with fluorescein. Br Med J 1962;ii:1210–1215.
14 Dollery CT, Hodge JV: Hypertensive retinopathy studies with fluorescein. Trans Ophthalmol Soc UK 1963;83:115–126.
15 Hodge JV, Dollery CT: Retinal soft exudates. Q J Med 1964;117–131.
16 Hill D: Fluorescence angiography. Trans Ophthalmol Soc UK 1968;88:187–189.
17 Gass JDM: A fluorescein angiographic study of macular dysfunction secondary to retinal vascular disease. III. Hypertensive retinopathy. Arch Ophthalmol 1968;80:569–582.
18 Garner A. Experimental Hypertensive Retinopathy; PhD Thesis, London, 1972.
19 Garner A, Ashton N, Tripathi R, et al. Pathogenesis of hypertensive retinopathy: An experimental study in the monkey. Br J Ophthalmol 1975;59:3–44.
20 Hayreh SS, Servais GE, Virdi PS: Retinal arteriolar changes in malignant arterial hypertension. Ophthalmologica 1989;198:178–196.
21 Hayreh SS, Servais GE, Virdi PS: Cotton-wool spots (Inner Retinal Ischemic Spots) in malignant arterial hypertension. Ophthalmologica 1989;198: 197–215.
22 Hayreh SS, Servais GE, Virdi PS: Macular lesions in malignant arterial hypertension. Ophthalmologica 1989;198:230–246.
23 Hayreh SS, Servais GE, Virdi PS: Retinal lipid deposits in malignant arterial hypertension. Ophthalmologica 1989;198:216–229.
24 Hayreh SS: Classification of hypertensive fundus changes and their order of appearance. Ophthalmologica 1989;198:247–260.
25 Hayreh SS, Servais GE: Retinal hemorrhages in malignant arterial hypertension. Int Ophthalmol 1988;12:137–145,197.
26 Hogan MJ, Alvarado JA, Weddell JE: Histology of the Human Eye: An Atlas and Textbook. Philadelphia, Saunders, 1971, pp 508–513.
27 Friedenwald JS, Wilder HC, Maumenee AE, et al. Ophthalmic Pathology, an Atlas and Textbook. Philadelphia, Saunders, 1952, p 310.
28 Malmfors T: The adrenergic innervation of the eye as demonstrated by fluorescence microscopy. Acta Physiol Scand 1965;65:259–267.
29 Ehinger B: Adrenergic nerves to the eye and to related structures in man and in the cynomolgus monkey *(Macaca irus)*. Invest Ophthalmol 1966; 5:42–52.
30 Laties AM: Central retinal artery innervation: Absence of adrenergic innervation to the intraocular branches. Arch Ophthalmol 1967;77:405–409.
31 Furukawa H: Autonomic innervation of preretinal blood vessels of the rabbit. Invest Ophthalmol Vis Sci 1987;28:1752–1760.
32 Porsaa K: Experimental studies on the vasomotor innervation of the retinal arteries. Acta Ophthalmol 1941 (suppl 18).
33 Dollery CT, Hill DW, Hodge JV: The response of normal retinal blood vessels to angiotensin and noradrenaline. J Physiol 1963;165:500–507.
34 Russell RWR: Observations on intracerebral aneurysms. Brain 1963;86:425–442.
35 Alm A, Bill A: The oxygen supply to the retina. II. Effects of high intraocular pressure and of increased arterial carbon dioxide tension on uveal and retinal blood flow in cats; a study with radioactively labelled microspheres including flow determinations in brain and some other tissues. Acta Physiol Scand 1972;84:306–319.
36 Alm A, Bill A: Ocular and optic nerve blood flow at normal and increased intraocular pressures in monkeys *(Macaca irus)*: a study with radioactively labelled microspheres including flow determinations

in brain and some other tissues. Exp Eye Res 1973;15:15–29.
37 Bill A: Effects of acetazolamide and carotid occlusion on the ocular blood flow in unanesthetized rabbits. Invest Ophthalmol 1974;13:954–958.
38 Strandgaard S, Jones JV, MacKenzie ET, Harper AM: Upper limit of cerebral blood flow autoregulation in experimental renovascular hypertension in the baboon. Circ Res 1975;37:164–167.
39 Jones JV, Fitch W, MacKenzie ET, et al: Lower limit of cerebral blood flow autoregulation in experimental renovascular hypertension in the baboon. Circ Res 1976;39:555–557.
40 Shakib M, Cunha-Vaz JG: Studies on the permeability of the blood-retinal barrier. IV. Junctional complexes of the retinal vessels and their role in the permeability of the blood-retinal barrier. Exp Eye Res 1966;5:229–234.
41 Cunha-Vaz JG: Studies on the permeability of the blood-retinal barrier. III. Breakdown of the blood-retinal barrier by circulatory disturbances. Br J Ophthalmol 1966;50:505–516.

Dr. S. S. Hayreh
Department of Ophthalmology
University of Iowa
Hospitals and Clinics
Iowa City, IA 52242 (USA)

Ophthalmologica 1989;198:178–196

Retinal Arteriolar Changes in Malignant Arterial Hypertension

Sohan Singh Hayreh, Gary E. Servais, Prem Singh Virdi

Department of Ophthalmology University of Iowa, Iowa City, Iowa, USA

Key Words. Arterial hypertension · Arteriolar sclerosis · Arteriolar spasm · Blood pressure · Cotton-wool spots · Hypertensive retinopathy · Malignant arterial hypertension · Retina · Retinal arterioles

Abstract. Experimental renovascular malignant arterial hypertension was produced by modified Goldblatt's procedures, in 60 rhesus monkeys, and various retinal arteriolar changes in hypertensive retinopathy were studied in detail (by serial ophthalmoscopy, and stereoscopic color fundus photography and fluorescein fundus angiography on long-term follow-up). The retinal arteriolar changes, in ophthalmoscopically visible arterioles, consisted of arteriolar sclerosis and associated changes, e.g., increased arteriolar tortuosity, arteriolar narrowing and in some animals occlusion and sheathing of the fine arterioles; we could find no evidence of localized or generalized 'spasm' in these retinal arterioles. Eyes in animals with accelerated arterial hypertension revealed focal dilatation and leakage of the retinal precapillary terminal arterioles (resulting in development of focal intraretinal periarteriolar transudates), and also occlusion of the terminal retinal arterioles (producing cotton-wool spots and associated intraretinal microvascular abnormalities). We discuss the controversial subjects of narrowing (particularly 'spasm') of ophthalmoscopically visible retinal arterioles and of fibrinoid necrosis in malignant hypertension.

Retinal arteriolar changes in malignant arterial hypertension have been mentioned in practically every publication on the subject since the first description of 'albuminuric retinitis' by Liebreich [1] in 1859. Almost all the classifications of hypertensive retinopathy have been based essentially on retinal arteriolar changes. A huge volume of literature has accumulated on the subject; nevertheless, the subject of retinal arteriolar changes in malignant hypertension is still controversial. Almost all the clinically available information on the subject is drawn from ophthalmoscopic examination of patients, most having chronic benign hypertension, and very little from studies in patients with malignant hypertension. Retinal arteriolar narrowing in hypertensive retinopathy has been described as the essential change, and Gowers [2], in 1876, first attributed this narrowing to arterial hypertension. The major focus of contention concerning retinal arteriolar changes in malignant hypertension has been the presence or absence of 'spasm' of retinal arterioles on ophthalmoscopy. Volhard and Fahr [3], in 1914, called it 'angiospastic retinopathy', and they [4, 5] seem to have been the first to advance the idea that narrowing of retinal arterioles in hypertension is due to spasm; this has since become classical teaching, advocated as an essential criterion in the diagnosis and classification of hypertensive retinopathy. Stokoe and Turner [6], by contrast, stressed that 'the frequently quoted sign of diffuse narrowing of the retinal arterioles as an early manifestation of hypertension is unreliable'. Similarly, Nicholls et al. [7] concluded that arteriolar caliber changes are not a good index of the degree of hypertension nor of the time it has existed. Cogan [8] stated that spasm seems unlikely because of the small amount of muscle in the retinal arterioles, the absence of any visible changes in the narrowing over a reasonable period of time, and the histologic evidence of hyalinization; he further added that 'Over-interpreting arterial narrowing in the fundus is a common failing. When one knows the patient has hypertension, one tends to attach undue significance to questionable changes'. The other argument put forward against spasm causing retinal segmental narrowing has been that when the blood pressure (BP) returns to normal after treatment, such areas rarely change their appearance and can even be seen in postmortem specimens. Moore [9] in 1917 showed that local retinal arteriolar narrowing was due to histologic changes in the vessel wall. Pickering [10], an authority on arterial hypertension, considered retinal arteriolar narrowing to be due to organic changes, and he stated that 'so far as human observations are concerned, this problem [of retinal arteriolar spasm] may now be said to be dead'. Dollery [11] mentioned the presence of focal and generalized narrowing of the larger retinal arterioles and irregularity of the smaller vessels in malignant hypertension, but also added that the larger arterioles are sometimes wide, tortuous, and irregular. This is just a quick overview of the extensive controversy on the topic of 'spasm' of the ophthalmoscopically seen retinal arterioles.

Modern investigative techniques [2, 12–18] have helped greatly to improve our understanding of this condition. In this paper we shall describe and discuss, in the light of our experimental studies, the various hypertensive retinal arteriolar changes seen in malignant arterial hypertension *(but not in benign arterial hypertension)*, as well as some major controversies on the subject.

Materials and Methods

Renovascular malignant arterial hypertension was produced in 60 rhesus monkeys by a modified Goldblatt's procedure. Details of the methods employed in this study to produce malignant arterial hypertension and evaluation of blood pressure and fundus changes are reported elsewhere [19]. Briefly, the animals consisted of two groups: a *one-kidney, one-clip model* (25 monkeys) which had only one kidney, and that kidney was ischemic, and a *two-kidney, one-clip model* (35 monkeys) which had one ischemic and one normal kidney. All monkeys were investigated by recording renal function, BP and fundus changes (by direct and indirect ophthalmoscopy, and stereoscopic color fundus photography and fluorescein fundus angiography) before renal artery clamping and serially thereafter. The method of recording BP in this experimental monkey model is discussed at length elsewhere [19]; we could reliably record only the systolic BP. To record the evolution of the BP and fundus changes, the various follow-up procedures were performed much more frequently during the initial acute stages, and less frequently later during the chronic phase (depending upon the severity of BP and the fundus changes). The frequency of the procedures also depended very much on the health of the monkey, because fundus photography and fluorescein fundus angiography, and the nembutal general anesthesia required for these procedures, are highly stressful to a sick, hypertensive monkey. Thus the follow-up for each animal was individualized to obtain the best possible information without detriment to the survival of the animal.

BP and ophthalmoscopic and fluorescein fundus angiographic findings on retinal arteriolar changes and other retinal lesions for all the monkeys were evaluated critically during the longitudinal follow-up period. The data for each animal were tabulated for retinal arteriolar changes (separately for one-kidney and two-kidney models), for various parameters, e.g., time since renal artery clamping, BP, and all retinal and fundus lesions.

We were specifically interested in the narrowing ('spasm') of the ophthalmoscopically visible moderate-to-large retinal arterioles in malignant arterial hypertension, since almost all previous accounts of ophthalmoscopic findings in this disease strongly stress it as an early and diagnostic feature of malignant arterial hypertension. To determine whether there was any (segmental or generalized) 'spasm' of the retinal arterioles in our animals with malignant arterial hypertension, we compared the width of the lumen of the major retinal arterioles (as seen on fluorescein fundus angiograms), in all animals, before renal artery clamping and after, through the entire hypertensive phase.

The data were finally collated and analyzed separately for the two models. The median (the 50th percentage point in data) and interquartile range (IQR; the difference between the 75th and 25th percentage points) are presented for most of the parameters, because these statistics present a better picture of the center and spread of a distribution than do the mean and standard deviation when there are extreme values in the data, as was mostly the case in this study. The Wilcoxon rank sum test and Spearman correlation coefficient were used to determine the statistical significances.

Results

BP, Hypertensive Retinopathy and Follow-Up Period

Table 1 summarizes the data on the BP, incidence of hypertensive retinopathy and length of follow-up. The normal median systolic BP in rhesus monkeys was 120 (with IQR 15) mm Hg. We decided to consider a systolic BP of 160 mm Hg or greater as hypertensive. Detailed general BP findings are reported elsewhere [19]. Renovascular hypertension developed in all 60 monkeys. It developed significantly ($p = 0.01$) earlier in the one-kidney than in the two-kidney model; however, there was no significant difference either in the time it took for the BP to reach its one-time highest recorded level or in the one-time peak recorded BP, between the two models [19]. Five of the 25 one-kidney monkeys died within 3 weeks after renal artery clamping from complications of accelerated hypertension or uremia. Some evidence of hypertensive retinopathy developed in 19 one-kidney monkeys (out of the 20 surviving 3≥ weeks) and 19 of the 35 two-kidney monkeys.

Retinal Arteriolar Changes

In the One-Kidney Model. Retinal arterioles developed changes in 13 of the 19 animals in this group which developed hypertensive retinopathy.

(1) The first arteriolar change: this was documented 29–407 (median 97, IQR 57) days after the renal artery clamping, after arterial hypertension for 22–402 (median 92, IQR 65) days, and maximum BP during this period was 190–240 (median 210, IQR 18) mm Hg. There was a significant correlation ($p \leq 0.005$) between the *duration* of arterial hypertension (but not the *level*) and the time it took to develop first detectable retinal arteriolar change. The first arteriolar change comprised: (a) early arteriolar sclerosis (which included abnormal light reflex, irregular width, and increased tortuosity of arterioles, and arteriovenous crossing changes) (in 8); (b) slightly increased arteriolar tortuosity (in 6 of the animals with reti-

Table 1. Length of follow-up, BP findings and hypertensive retinopathy in one-kidney and two-kidney animals

	One-kidney group (25 monkeys)			Two-kidney group (35 monkeys)		
	range	median	IQR	range	median	IQR
Follow-up period, months	1.2–57.3[1]	9.6[1]	19.2[1]	0.7–42.3	26.4	10.5
Time interval (days) from renal artery clamping to						
Onset of hypertension	2– 43	7	3	2–115	15	18
Maximum BP recorded	2–980	110	287	8–899	124	237
Onset of hypertensive retinopathy	12– 63[2]	22[2]	17[2]	8–302[3]	64[3]	44[3]
Highest BP recorded						
BP level, in mm Hg	178–260	220	30	160–260	204	50
% Rise from baseline BP	148–245	193	46	133–237	175	26
BP at onset of hypertensive retinopathy, mm Hg	164–225[2]	190[2]	21[2]	160–210[3]	178[3]	26[3]

1 In 20 animals that survived ≥3 weeks.
2 Hypertensive retinopathy seen in 19 one-kidney monkeys.
3 Hypertensive retinopathy seen in 19 two-kidney monkeys.

nal arteriolar sclerotic changes); (c) slight attenuation of the arterioles (in 4), and (d) occlusion and sheathing of one of the fine arterioles (in 1 eye). At this stage, in these one-kidney eyes, the retinopathy varied from mild to marked (usually moderate) in severity, and there was no difference in the severity of retinopathy in animals with and without arteriolar changes. No retinal arteriolar changes developed in the remaining 5 animals, during a follow-up of 26 to >1,000 (median 68, IQR 162) days, with arterial hypertension lasting for a median period of 56 (IQR 160) days and a maximum BP of 175–240 (median 225, IQR 14) mm Hg.

(2) Arteriolar changes on follow-up: the 13 animals with retinal arteriolar changes showed the following alterations: (a) increased tortuosity, usually of mild degree, in all the animals, 61–407 (median 153.5, IQR 75) days after renal artery clamping (fig. 1, 2); (b) arteriolar sclerotic change, in 12 animals in 61–364 (median 105, IQR 90) days (fig. 1, 2); (c) arteriolar narrowing of mild to marked degree, in 9 animals in 23–497 (median 104, IQR 259) days; (d) a few of the fine retinal arterioles developed complete occlusion and sheathing in 10 animals, 56–308 (median 160, IQR 119) days after renal artery clamping (fig. 1c, d, 2). The sheathing and occlusion were almost always located at the posterior pole, mostly involving the small arterioles arising from the main temporal retinal arterioles and supplying the macular region, and only rarely at other sites in the posterior retina. These developments were

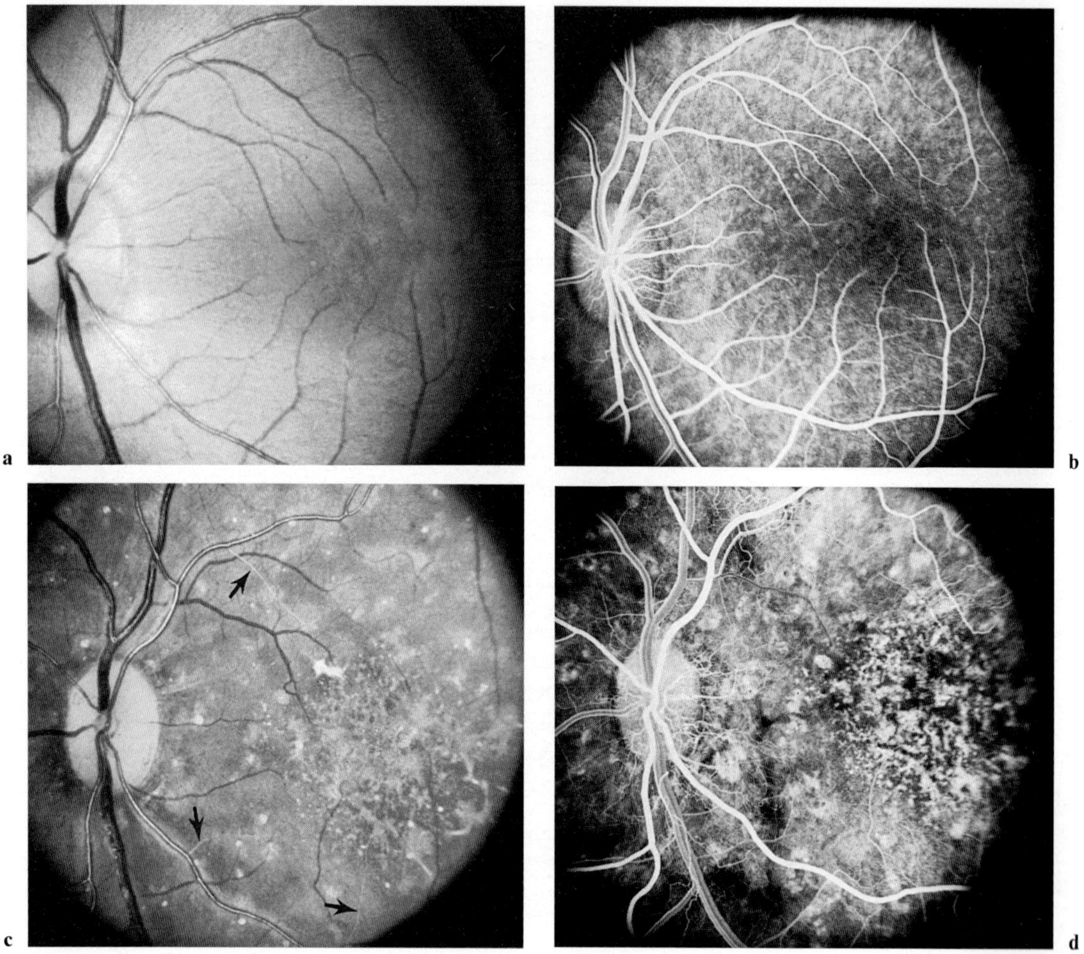

Fig. 1. Fundus photographs (**a, c**) and fluorescein fundus angiograms (**b, d**) of left eye of a one-kidney model monkey before Goldblatt's procedure (**a, b**) and 354 days (BP 220 mm Hg) thereafter (**c, d**). **a, b** Normal fundus and angiogram. **c** Fundus photograph shows retinal arteriolar sclerosis, increased arteriolar tortuosity and sheathing of fine arterioles (arrows), intraretinal microvascular abnormalities, retinal atrophy, and focal and macular retinal pigment epithelial degenerative changes; compare the state of the retinal vessels and of the fundus background in **c** with that in **a. d** Angiogram, during the retinal arteriovenous phase, shows extensive retinal capillary obliteration, occlusion of the sheathed retinal arterioles and widely scattered retinal pigment epithelial degenerative changes; note the angiographic changes as compared to the normal in **b**.

related to capillary obliteration due to cotton-wool spots (CWSs) [20]. The number of these sheathed and occluded arterioles progressively increased with time, as also did retinal capillary obliteration [20].

In the Two-Kidney Model. Appreciable retinal arteriolar changes were seen in only 5 animals. These included sheathing of the retinal arterioles in the macular region, associated with CWSs and retinal capillary obliteration,

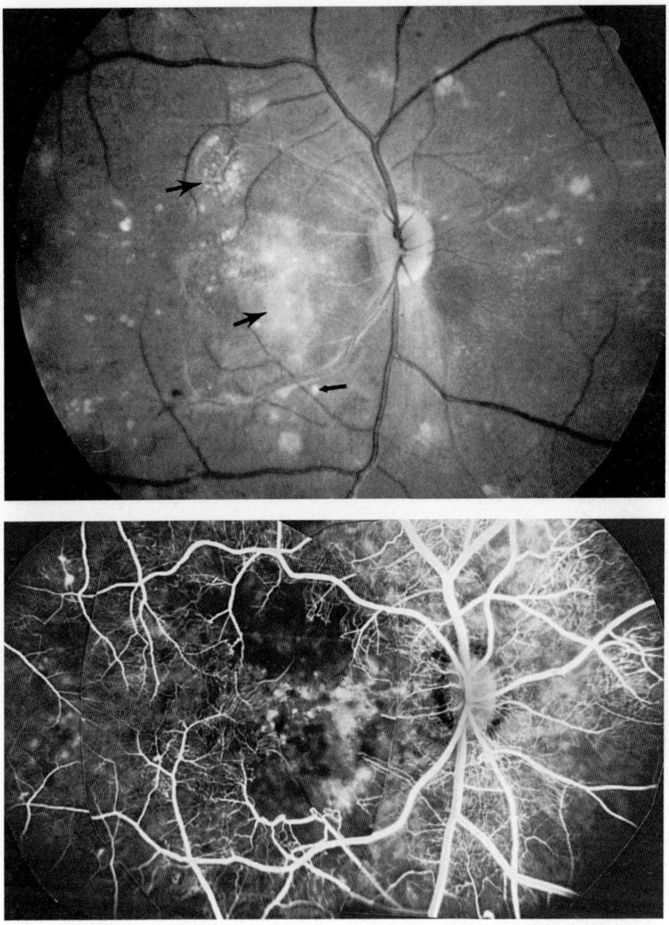

a

b

Fig. 2. Ophthalmoscopic and fluorescein angiographic appearance of right eye of a one-kidney monkey (day 293; BP 204 mm Hg). **a** Fundus photograph shows arteriolar sclerosis with marked narrowing of retinal arterioles, sheathing of small arterioles, a few fine lipid deposits, resolving CWSs (large arrows), occasional FIPT (small arrow), and focal and macular retinal pigment epithelial degenerative lesions, and flat macular retinal detachment with a subretinal exudative veil. **b** Angiogram, during the retinal arteriovenous phase, shows normal caliber of the arterioles, occlusion of the sheathed arterioles, extensive retinal capillary obliteration in the posterior pole and some intraretinal microvascular abnormalities.

in 3 animals, developing about 4, 18 and 24 months respectively after the renal artery clamping and about 1, 15 and 21 months, respectively, after the start of development of CWSs, all of which were marked. Three animals revealed mild arteriolar sclerotic change 2–7 months after the onset of hypertension. However, other animals in this group with raised BP lasting for even longer did not have such arteriolar change. *The overall degree of sustained rise of BP in the two-kidney animals was much lower than in the one-kidney monkeys, although one-time peak BP recorded was no different in the two models.*

'Spasm' of Retinal Arterioles during the Acute Phase of Malignant Arterial Hypertension

During the acute phase of malignant arterial hypertension, we could find no fluorescein angiographically demonstrable localized or generalized arteriolar narrowing ('spasm') in any animal (either the one-kidney or the two-kidney), in spite of a very high, sustained BP.

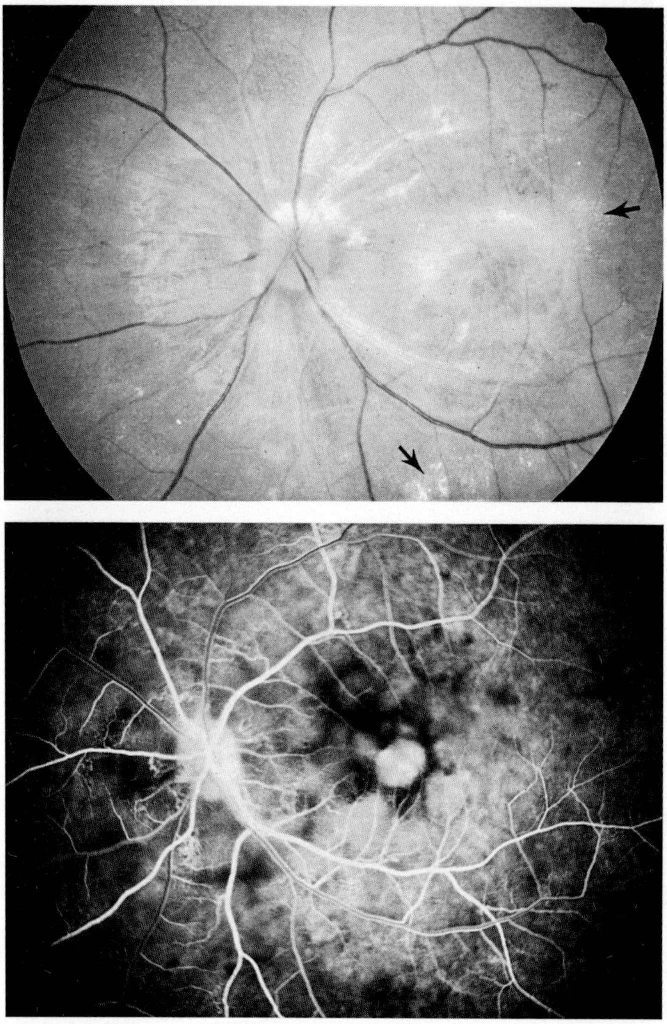

a

b

Fig. 3. Ophthalmoscopic and fluorescein angiographic appearance of left eye of a one-kidney monkey (day 251; BP 220 mm Hg). **a** Fundus photograph shows marked attenuation of the retinal arterioles all over, with retinal edema, microcystic macular edema, serous retinal detachment and subretinal exudative deposits in the macular region and a few lipid deposits (arrows). **b** Angiogram, during the early retinal arteriovenous phase, shows normal caliber of the retinal arterioles, patches of delayed filling of the choroidal vascular bed, patchy unmasking of the submacular choroidal fluorescence, and patches of retinal capillary nonperfusion.

Although on ophthalmoscopy many eyes showed an apparent narrowing of the retinal arterioles, on fluorescein fundus angiography no change in size from the baseline lumen width could be detected. Our fluorescein fundus angiographic findings showed that the apparent retinal arteriolar narrowing (generalized or segmental) in these eyes was an ophthalmoscopic artifact – '*pseudo-narrowing*'; to illustrate this important new fact, we present here 6 examples from our one-kidney series (fig. 2–6). Once the arteriolar sclerotic changes developed, of course, the retinal arterioles showed a variable degree of arteriolar narrowing – but that is very different from the 'spasm' during the acute phase stressed in the literature.

In a few eyes, when the BP was very high (in 1 animal between 225 and 240 mm Hg), the

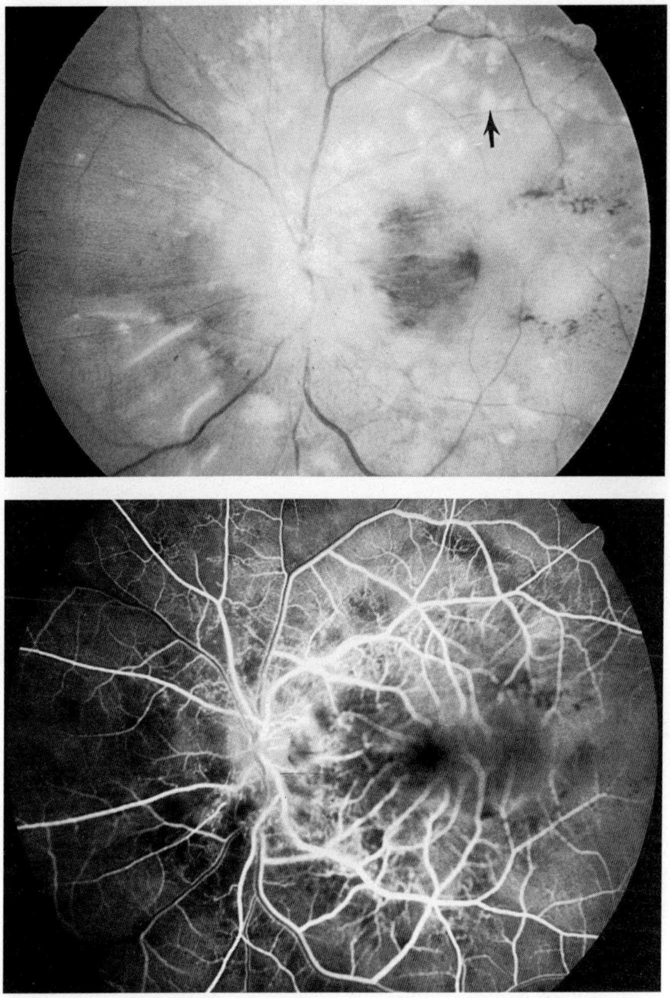

a

b

Fig. 4. Ophthalmoscopic (**a**) and fluorescein angiographic (**b**) appearance of left eye of a one-kidney monkey on day 42 (BP 200 mm Hg; this was inadvertently reported as 164 mm Hg in a previous publication [21a]). **a** Fundus photograph shows marked attenuation of the retinal arterioles, retinal and macular edema, multiple FIPTs (arrow), retinal hemorrhages and extensive serous retinal detachment with thick exudative subretinal fluid in the macular region. **b** On the same day angiogram, during the retinal early arteriovenous phase, shows normal caliber of the retinal arterioles, with delayed filling of the choroid posteriorly. Published courtesy of *Ophthalmology* 1986;93:60–73 [21a].

entire arteriolar tree of the major retinal arterioles showed pulsation.

Comment

The so-called 'retinal arteries' seen on ophthalmoscopy are, anatomically, arterioles. The retinal vascular bed has the properties of autoregulation [21a] and blood-retinal barrier [21a] but it has no autonomic nerve supply. These basic anatomic and physiologic properties of the retinal vessels may play an important role in the production of various retinal arteriolar changes.

Fluorescein fundus angiography provides essential information on several important aspects of the retinal arteriolar bed, including

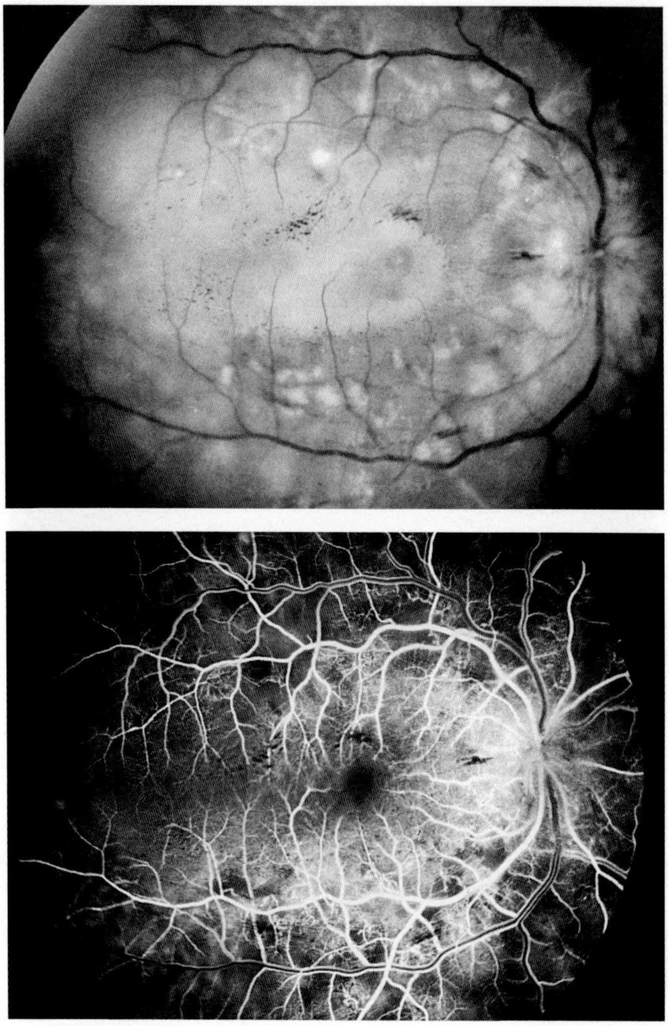

a

b

Fig. 5. Ophthalomoscopic (**a**) and fluorescein angiographic (**b**) appearance of right eye of a one-kidney monkey (day 64; BP 198 mm Hg). **a** Fundus photograph shows marked attenuation of retinal arterioles, macular and retinal edema, foveal cyst, serous retinal detachment of macular region with exudative opaque subretinal fluid, and other hypertensive retinal lesions. Published courtesy of *Ophthalmology* 1986;93:1383–1400 [21b]. **b** Angiogram, during retinal early arteriovenous phase, shows normal caliber of the retinal arterioles and patches of retinal capillary non-perfusion corresponding to the CWSs.

the arteriolar caliber, patency or obliteration, state of the blood-retinal barrier, and blood flow. In addition, it also shows the retinal vessels as wider than ophthalmoscopy or color photographs do. This is because in the retinal arterioles, as elsewhere in the blood vessels, the cells in the blood concentrate in the axial stream, with the peripheral part of the blood column carrying mainly plasma; since fluorescein mixes in the plasma, fluorescein fundus angiography reveals the entire width of the blood column, whereas ophthalmoscopy and color fundus photography show only the width of the central column of red blood cells. It is important to understand this discrepancy between the angiographic and ophthalmoscopic findings. The information in the literature on the retinal arteriolar changes in hypertensive

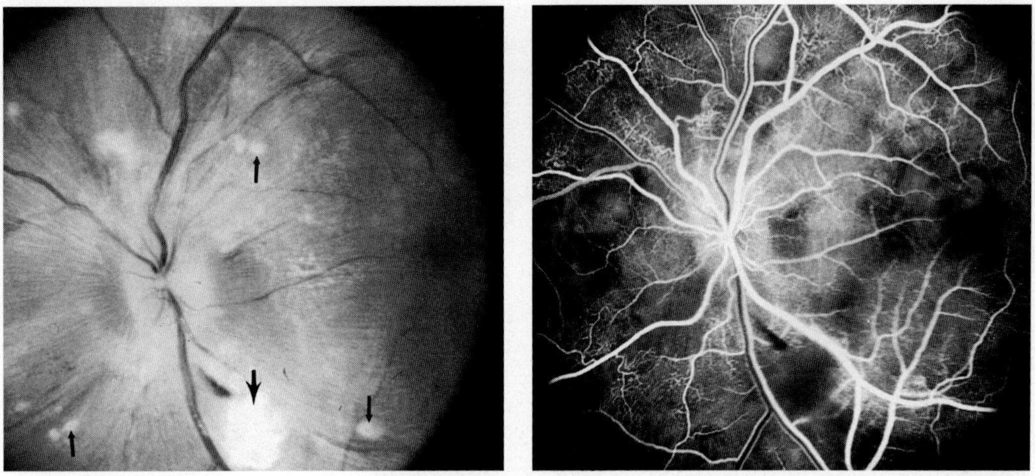

a b

Fig. 6. Ophthalmoscopic and fluorescein angiographic appearance of a one-kidney monkey: left eye (**a, b**) on day 63 (BP 192 mm Hg), and right eye (**c, d**) on day 78 (BP 190 mm Hg). **a** Fundus photograph shows multiple FIPTs (small arrows), CWSs (large arrow) and acute focal retinal pigment epithelial lesions, narrowing of retinal arterioles, macular edema and moderate macular serous retinal detachment. Published courtesy of *Ophthalmology* 1986;93:60–73 [21a]. **b** Angiogram, during retinal early arteriovenous phase, shows normal caliber of retinal arterioles, patches of retinal capillary non-perfusion (corresponding to active or resolved CWSs), and delayed choroidal filling.

retinopathy comes mainly from ophthalmoscopy or color fundus photography, and very little from fluorescein angiography. This may be one reason for the conflict between our findings and those in the literature; our study is the first detailed, systematic study of hypertensive retinopathy in rhesus monkeys to utilize frequent serial stereoscopic color fundus photography and fluorescein fundus angiography and correlation between them, with a long term follow-up.

'Spasm' of the Retinal Arterioles

As discussed earlier, 'spasm' of ophthalmoscopically seen retinal arterioles is said to be the classical change in arteriolar hypertension, and has been the major focus of contention in hypertensive retinopathy. In the retina, numerous muscle cells embrace the terminal arterioles and extend even as far as the precapillary arterioles where they gradually, indistinguishably merge with the pericytes of capillaries [22] so that the terminal arterioles are capable of contraction. Bayliss [23] demonstrated in 1902 that vascular smooth muscle will contract in response to stretching. Pal [24], 1905, attributed the local vascular disturbances in arterial hypertension to brief local arteriolar spasm provoked directly by excessive tension in the vessel, i.e. the Bayliss effect. Similarly, the retinal arteriolar 'spasm' in arterial hypertension has been attributed to the Bayliss effect [23–25]. Volhard [4, 5, 26] attributed the signs and symptoms of hypertension to a chronic form of spasm. Hypertensive retinopathy has therefore been classified by some as 'angiospastic retinopathy' [3, 27–29].

Based on their clinical observations, Wagener et al. [29] concluded that three distinct

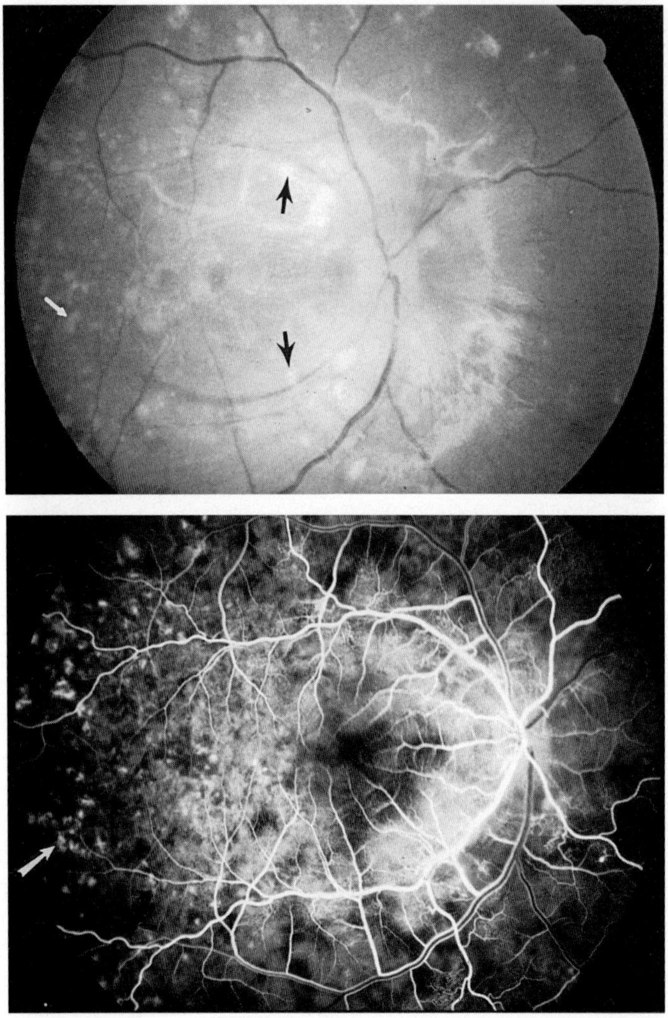

c

d

Fig. 6. **c** Fundus photograph shows extreme attenuation of retinal arterioles, microcystic macular edema, serous macular detachment with mostly clear and some exudative subretinal fluid, and multiple FIPTs (black arrows), and acute focal retinal pigment epithelial lesions (white arrow). **d** Angiogram, during retinal early arteriovenous phase, shows normal caliber of retinal arterioles, and punctate fluorescent spots (arrow) corresponding to the focal retinal pigment epithelial lesions.

types of change occur in the retinal arterioles in hypertension: (1) generalized narrowing, which, they felt, probably represented the generally increased tone of the arterioles; (2) sclerosis due to organic thickening of the wall, and (3) focal constriction ('spasm'). From this concept, they described the following arteriolar changes in hypertension: (a) generalized narrowing, (b) 'spasm' or focal constriction, (c) generalized sclerosis, (d) focal sclerosis, (e) sheathing, and (f) occlusion. They further added that in many cases of chronic hypertension, spasm is combined with, or superimposed on, arteriolar sclerosis. Leishman [30], in his classic clinical studies, stated that the degree of spasm ('hypertonus' response) in the retinal arterioles in hypertension depends upon the height of the BP and the degree of 'involutionary sclerosis' (replacement fibrosis); i.e. with raised intraluminal pressure, the normal segments become hypertonic (turning narrow, straight and pale), while the fibrotic segments dilate and lengthen passively (assuming a wide, red, curvilinear appearance). If the hypertensive stimulus is continued and is not too intense, reactive changes produce diffuse thickening of the arteriolar wall, resulting in a hyperplastic arteriole (having a narrow blood column with variable caliber, a markedly pale look, and, at the arteriovenous crossing, the arteriole hides the underlying vein). However, in malignant hypertension there is no time for replacement fibrosis, and hyperplasia proceeds to acute arteriolar necrosis. In less severe hypertension, fibrosis replaces hyperplasia in the arterioles. According to Leishman [30], since hypertonus merges into hyperplasia and that in turn into fibrosis, all three processes may occur simultaneously in different parts of the same arteriole. He further added that in malignant hypertension the arterioles look normal near the optic disc but 'in some portions the pallor is accentuated and the calibre of the blood column is reduced and finely variable'. Reversible narrowing of retinal arterioles in malignant hypertension has been alleged in a number of clinical studies [24, 26, 27, 31–37]. Ramalho and Dollery [37] found that on lowering the BP in hypertensive patients the small arterioles ($<50\,\mu m$) dilated, while medium and larger arterioles (50–$70\,\mu m$) usually remained unchanged.

Retinal arteriolar narrowing (localized and/or generalized) has also been reported in a large number of studies on experimental arterial hypertension, conducted mostly in rats [25, 38–44], with an odd one in rabbits [45], dogs [46] or monkeys [47]; this has been described in some reports as reversible narrowing [38, 40, 43, 46]. Narrowing and irregularity of the retinal arterioles have been attributed by some observers [9, 10, 48] – but not all [26, 27, 38, 46] – to progressive anatomic narrowing. Garner [17] and Garner et al. [18], by contrast, in experimental malignant hypertension in cynomolgus monkeys, found no focal or generalized narrowing of retinal arterioles, on either ophthalmoscopy or fluorescein fundus angiography; they found the main retinal arterioles, if anything, dilated and tortuous, particularly in severer hypertensive retinopathy.

Limitations of the Findings in the Literature

In the evaluation of narrowing of retinal arterioles in patients with arterial hypertension, a number of factors can result in misleading information. These include subjective ophthalmoscopic criteria, combined with preconceived notions and no controls; overinterpretation of retinal arteriolar narrowing in patients known to be hypertensive (as pointed out by Cogan [8]); lumping together of cases of benign and malignant hypertension; arteriolar sclerosis due to aging confused with changes due to hypertension; use of the arteriovenous ratio to judge the narrowing, and many more. For example, the arteriovenous ratio on ophthalmoscopic fundus examination has been used as a standard method to evaluate retinal arteriolar narrowing in hypertension and other conditions, but this method has been shown to be highly deceptive [6, 49–51], with an intraobserver disagreement of $33\pm12\%$ and interobserver disagreement of $42\pm17\%$ [50]. Thus, in considering the controversy on retinal arteriolar narrowing in malignant arterial hypertension, one has to bear in mind these various limitations as well as a number of other factors, all of which seem to confuse the issue. For instance, the term 'spasm' itself has been used ambiguously by ophthalmologists. It must be stressed that *tone* is a sustained physiological contraction whereas *spasm* is a sudden strong abnormal contraction for a limited period only; thus we cannot have 'spasm' of the arterioles going on for months. Aging arteriolar sclerosis, arteriolar hyperplasia in benign chronic hypertension and 'spasm' have all been confused with one another.

In the limited number of fluorescein fundus angiographic studies available on malignant hypertension in patients in the literature, it was frequently stated that there was narrowing of the retinal arterioles, but a careful review by us of published angiograms did not reveal any appreciable narrowing in the vast majority, although such narrowing or irregular lumen was seen in eyes with chronic hypertension with arteriolar sclerosis.

Stenosis of the terminal arterioles in malignant hypertension is well established, and there is ample clinical and pathological evidence of it in the various organs. It is of fundamental importance to realize that hypertensive retinopathy is essentially a manifestation of vascular disturbance at the level of the *precapillary retinal arterioles,* and Ashton [52] rightly pointed out that these vessels are too small to be seen ophthalmoscopically. It is the contraction of ophthalmoscopically visible larger retinal arterioles which has been described by various workers in hypertension. One has to bear in mind that the amount of constriction of these large arterioles attributable to hypertension, if any, is so small that it cannot make any appreciable hemodynamic difference to the retinal circulation. Thus, whether there is a slight narrowing of the ophthalmoscopically visible retinal arterioles or not is totally irrelevant to our understanding of the pathogenesis of the various lesions in hypertensive retinopathy; anyway, this is too subjective a criterion to be useful in diagnosis. Yet controversy on the subject continues, generating a good deal more heat than light!

In view of this, one of the major objectives of the present study was to evaluate the retinal arteriolar narrowing at different stages of arterial hypertension in our monkey model. For the reasons discussed above, we were specifically interested in the vasospastic narrowing of the ophthalmoscopically visible retinal arterioles during the initial phase of malignant hypertension. We could find no generalized or focal narrowing of these arterioles in any of our monkeys with severe malignant hypertension. Although many eyes with hypertensive retinopathy and retinal edema showed pseudo-narrowing of the retinal arterioles in color fundus photographs and on ophthalmoscopy, fluorescein fundus angiography revealed no real narrowing of these arterioles at all when compared to the baseline prehypertension angiograms (fig. 2–6). Evidently in our series the ophthalmoscopically seen narrowing was due to retinal edema masking a part of the vessel, producing pseudo-narrowing. This absence of retinal arteriolar narrowing on angiography even with very high BP was totally unexpected. Such an absence of narrowing has also been reported in monkeys in excellent studies by Garner and coworkers [17, 18, 52]. Most studies in rats and dogs have reported retinal arteriolar narrowing all the time. It is hard to give a definite reason for this discrepancy. It could be argued that this is a species difference, with rats responding differently from monkeys. Yet all the available evidence indicates that anatomically and physiologically the retinal vascular bed of rhesus monkeys behaves very much like that of man, so that our observations and those of Garner and coworkers [17, 18, 52] should be applicable to man as well. We can only repeat that in the present study, during the acute phase of malignant arterial hypertension, the major retinal arterioles and their subdivisions (visible on ophthalmoscopy) showed no generalized or focal contraction on fluorescein angiography. Could a marked fall in BP under deep nembutal anesthesia, required for fundus photography and fluorescein fundus angiography, have abolished the arteriolar spasm, as suggested by a number of authors [40, 43, 53, 54]? We measured the BP in our hypertensive monkeys just before and during nembutal anesthesia, and there was a mean fall of only 5.7±3.9 (SD) mm Hg or 3.4% in systolic BP – too small a drop to account for our not finding arteriolar spasm. Moreover, the pseudo-narrowing of the retinal arterioles was present on ophthalmoscopy and color fundus photographs at the time when fluorescein fundus angiography revealed a normal caliber in the arterioles. Late in the disease, however, when arteriolar sclerotic changes supervened, we did see a variable degree of narrowing in the retinal arterioles.

We want to stress strongly that the retinal arteriolar findings of the present study are applicable basically to *malignant hypertension*. Whether and to what extent these retinal arteriolar findings are also valid in chronic essential hypertension of low grade in man remains unknown. We did not study that aspect; we are currently studying just that in a large colony of rhesus monkeys with chronic mild arterial hypertension, over a period of several years.

Other Retinal Arteriolar Changes

These include the following:

Focal Dilatation and Leakage of Precapillary Terminal Retinal Arterioles (FIPTs). During the acute phase of accelerated arterial hypertension, because of the severe rise of BP, dilatation of these arterioles is produced by failure of autoregulation [21a]. The dilatation results in breakdown of blood-retinal barrier in the involved arterioles. These lesions lead to the formation of FIPTs (discussed by us at length previously [21a].

Occlusion of the Terminal Retinal Arterioles. This results in the production of CWSs (inner retinal ischemic spots), which are discussed in detail elsewhere [20]. A few of the fine arterioles at the posterior pole also developed complete occlusion and sheathing in the distribution of CWSs, usually related to retinal capillary obliteration [20] (fig. 1, 2). Garner [17] and Garner et al. [18], in experimental malignant hypertension in monkeys, also found closure of precapillary retinal arterioles as the most striking morphologic feature.

Fibrinoid Necrosis of Arterioles. This is considered the most characteristic pathological feature of arteriolar changes in malignant hypertension. Fibrin is deposited in the wall of small arteries and arterioles, due to passage of plasma proteins into the wall. Hence it is also called 'fibrinous vasculosis'. The pathogenesis of how and why plasma proteins gain entry to the vessel's wall still remains controversial, particularly in the retinal circulation where the tight cell junctions in the vascular endothelial cell are impervious to proteins. The passage of fibrin and lipid into the vessel wall has been stated to be through a damaged and leaking endothelium [55], the damage to the endothelium being attributed to the hypertension. Kincaid-Smith [56] proposed the following schema for the various vascular changes seen in malignant arterial hypertension: increase of endogenous vasoconstrictor agents (angiotensin, vasopressin, epinephrine) → 'sausage string' effect in arteries → turbulence and endothelial separation and damage → platelet deposition on endothelium → release of thromboxane, serotonin, histamine → microangiopathic hemolytic anemia and intravascular coagulation → further platelet and fibrin deposition → mitogenic and migration factors released by platelet aggregation → myointimal proliferation and organization of thrombi within vessels → renal ischemia → increase in vasoactive agents; thus a vicious circle is set up in malignant hypertension. Therefore, the primary process may be endothelial damage.

Garner and coworkers [17, 18, 52] have admirably reviewed the subject in the light of their excellent experimental and pathologic studies on hypertensive retinopathy. They postulated that the process of plasmatic vasculosis in the retina can be divided into four stages: in the *first stage* there is severe and unrelieved arteriolar constriction in the precapillary arterioles, resulting in virtual abolition of the lumen. The *second stage* consists of consequent ischemic degeneration of the contracted arteriolar smooth muscle. During the *third stage* there is atonic relaxation of the constriction because of degeneration of the muscle cells, and this is followed by focal rupture of the endothelial cell lining following restoration of blood flow through the arteriole. In the *fourth stage,* plasma proteins leak into the vessel wall through a defective endothelium, so that the wall becomes thickened and the lumen constricts again. They felt that selective muscle necrosis in the arterioles cannot be explained by anything other than ischemia secondary to obliteration of the vessel lumen. However, Giese [57] postulated that muscle necrosis can be secondary to fibrinous insudation.

The studies by Garner and coworkers [17, 18, 52], while very meticulously done, pose some serious problems with their observations and interpretations. Some of the difficulties we have with these studies include the following:

(a) If arteriolar spasm was the primary factor in initiating the process, as postulated by them, then why was no extensive capillary nonperfusion revealed by fluorescein angiography at that stage in their study? They did consider the possibility that the obliteration of the arterioles seen on electron microscopy could have been a postenucleation fixation artifact, but felt that this was not likely.

(b) In our studies on FIPTs [21a], we found leakage of the dye (and the proteins) through the wall of terminal retinal arterioles (also clearly shown by our recent histopathologic studies), without any evidence of their occlusion on fluorescein angiography before, at that time or later; this conflicts with the speculation by Garner [17], Garner et al. [18] and Ashton [52] on their fourth stage mentioned above.

(c) In the pathogenesis of 'CWSs', these authors speculated that ischemic damage to the related area of the nerve fiber layer occurred during the initial functional contraction phase, so that by the time the 'CWSs' were clinically established, the arterioles might be in a state of atonic dilatation and giving rise to exudation. This is because they found normal capillary filling in what they presumed were CWSs (these lesions in fact had all the feature of FIPTs).

These studies [17, 18, 52] were done by a collaboration of ocular pathologists (Garner, Ashton and Tripathi) and clinicians (dealing with fluorescein fundus angiography – Kohner, Bulpitt and Dollery). The latter group, being unaware of the existence of FIPTs, mistakenly considered them 'soft exudates' (they used this term synonymously for 'CWSs' in most of their publications) in this and in their previous studies on hypertensive retinopathy [13–15]. Our studies have shown that the FIPT is an exudative lesion situated in the deeper layers of the retina, with focal fluorescein leakage from the terminal retinal arterioles which are dilated, and normal capillary prefusion in their distribution [21a] – this angiographic pattern was erroneously considered by Garner's clinical collaborators [17, 18, 52] to be that of 'soft exudates' (or 'CWSs'.). In contrast to the FIPTs, it is well-established that the CWS is an ischemic lesion, with evidence of closure of terminal retinal arterioles, capillary nonperfusion in their distribution, usually no fluorescein leakage and focal infarction of the superficial nerve fiber layer [20]. In order to clarify this controversy, one of us (SSH) personally discussed at length with Professor A. Garner (in December 1987) the discrepancies between the studies by Garner [17], Garner et al. [18] and Ashton [52] and the present one by us. It emerged from that discussion that their pathological interpretation and their hypothesis on the pathogenesis of hypertensive retinopathy was influenced by their clinical interpretation of the so-called 'soft exudates', which they interpreted to represent CWSs, and thus included in 'soft exudates' two totally different types of lesions, FIPTs (an exudative lesion [21a]), and CWS (an ischemic lesion [20], because they believed that the two represented a continuum, with the FIPT being a precursor of the CWS [12–15]. Our studies clearly showed that this is not the case [20, 21a]. This misinterpretation distorted the interpretation of the pathological findings, hence the hypothesis of hypertensive arteriolar changes, i.e. plasmatic vasculosis and CWSs. Professor Garner now feels that – in the light of our findings that FIPTs [21a] and CWSs [20] are two totally unrelated lesions – it would seem reasonable to speculate that spasm of the terminal arterioles may lead to thrombosis in the arterioles, which would then lead to permanent closure of the terminal arterioles and focal nonperfusion of the retinal capillaries in CWSs, without any leakage. The other difference between the study by Garner and coworkers [17, 18, 52] and the present study is the fact that the primary objective of the study by Garner's group was to analyze only *the early vascular changes in hypertensive retinopathy,* so that most of their animals were sacrificed before florid retinal disease had time to develop. In our study, by contrast, we followed the animals for months if not years, so that we have more detailed long-term information on the evolution of the various lesions in hypertensive retinopathy.

Retinal Arteriolar Sclerosis. This has been well-established as a change in arterial hypertension ever since Duke Carl of Bavaria [58] first demonstrated it in 1887, and Buechner [59] stated that 'hypertension breeds arteriosclerosis'. As described above, in the present study, after prolonged hypertension and later on in the evolution of the disease, the retinal arterioles commonly showed variable degrees of arteriolar sclerosis, attenuation and increased tortuosity, and a few of the fine arterioles even developed complete occlusion and sheathing (fig. 1, 2).

In the literature, 'arteriolar reflex change', 'copper-wire arteries', 'silver-wire arteries' and so on are frequently mentioned as signs of arterial hypertension. These terms are of little scientific validity, and Leishman [30] very appropriately remarked that 'recording of clinical signs, such as 'copper-wire' arteries, caliber variations, arteriovenous ratios, and the vagaries of the vascular light reflex, may become the self-imposed limit of legitimate clinical thought concerning the retinal vessels' in hypertension; he further added that these terms have been used by most ophthalmologists without 'a clear conception of the meaning of these appearances'. Thus they serve no useful purpose.

Conclusions

In malignant arterial hypertension, during the early acute phase, the retinal arterioles show changes essentially in the terminal retinal arterioles (either dilatation with leakage resulting in the formation of FIPTs, or occlusion, which produces CWSs), there is no appreciable narrowing or spasm in the major retinal arterioles, although the latter show ophthalmoscopically variable degrees of pseudo-narrowing, due to masking of the arterioles by retinal edema. In chronic arterial hypertension, there are retinal arteriolar sclerosis and associated retinal arteriolar changes.

Acknowledgments

We are grateful to Dr. Robert F. Woolson and Dr. Marie R. Klugman of the Department of Preventive Medicine (Biostatistics) for their help with the statistical analyses of the data, to Mrs. Ellen Ballas and Mrs. Georgiane Parkes-Perret for their secretarial help, to Mr. James Swaner for the technical help, and to the Photography Department for the illustrations. This investigation was supported by a research grant from the National Eye Institute (EY-1576) and in part by an unrestricted grant from Research to Prevent Blindness, Inc., and from the Alcon Research Institute.

References

1 Liebreich R: Ophthalmoskopischer Befund bei Morbus Brightii. Graefes Arch Clin Exp Ophthalmol 1859;5:265–268.
2 Gowers WR: The state of the arteries in Bright's disease. Br Med J 1876;ii:743–745.
3 Volhard F, Fahr KT: Die Brightsche Nierenkrankheit: Klinik, Pathologie und Atlas, vol 8 Berlin, Springer, 1914.
4 Volhard F: Die Pathogenese der Retinitis albuminurica. Zentralbl Gesamte Opthalmol 1929;20:627–628.
5 Volhard F: Medizinischer Teil. Zentralbl Gesamte Ophthalmol 1921;5:470–481.
6 Stokoe NL, Turner RWD: Normal retinal vascular patterns. Arterio-venous ratio as measure of arterial calibre. Br J Ophthalmol 1966;50:21–40.
7 Nicholls JVV, Turnbull W, Evelyn KA: The calibre of the retinal arterioles in normal and hypertensive patients. Trans Can Ophthalmol Soc 1956;7:37–45.
8 Cogan DG: Ophthalmic Manifestations of Systemic Vascular Disease. Philadelphia, Saunders, 1974, pp 74–78.
9 Moore RF: The retinitis of arterio-sclerosis, and its relation to renal retinitis and to cerebral vascular disease. Q J Med 1917;10:29–77.
10 Pickering GW: High Blood Pressure, ed 2. London, Churchill, 1968, pp 342–343.
11 Dollery CT: Hypertensive retinopathy; in Genest J, Kuchel O, Hamet P et al (eds): Hypertension: Physiopathology and Treatment, ed 2. New York, McGraw-Hill 1983, pp 723–832.
12 Dollery CT, Hodge JV, Engel M: Studies of the retinal circulation with fluorescein. Br Med J 1962;ii:1210–1215.
13 Dollery CT, Hodge JV: Hypertensive retinopathy studied with fluorescein. Trans Ophthalmol Soc UK 1963;83:115–126.
14 Hodge JV, Dollery CT: Retinal soft exudates. Q J Med 1964;33:117–131.
15 Hill D: Fluorescence angiography. Trans Ophthalmol Soc UK 1968;88:187–189.
16 Gass JDM: A fluorescein angiographic study of macular dysfunction secondary to retinal vascular disease. III. Hypertensive retinopathy. Arch Ophthalmol 1968;80:569–582.
17 Garner A: Experimental Hypertensive Retinopathy; PhD thesis, London, 1972.
18 Garner A, Ashton N, Tripathi R, et al: Pathogenesis of hypertensive retinopathy: An experimental study in the monkey. Br J Ophthalmol 1975;59:3–44.
19 Hayreh SS, Servais GE, Virdi PS, et al: Fundus lesions in malignant hypertension. III. Arterial blood pressure, biochemical and fundus changes. Ophthalmology 1986;93:45–59.
20 Hayreh SS, Servais GE, Virdi PS: Cotton-wool spots (Inner retinal ischemic spots) in malignant arterial hypertension. Ophthalmologica 1989;198:197–215.
21a Hayreh SS, Servais GE, Virdi PS: Fundus lesions in malignant hypertension. IV. Focal intra-retinal periarteriolar transudates. Ophthalmology 1986;93:60–73.

21b Hayreh SS, Servais GE, Virdi PS: Fundus lesions in malignant hypertension. VI. Hypertensive choroidopathy. Ophthalmology 1986;93:1383–1400.
22 Ashton N, Harry H: The pathology of cotton-wool spots and cytoid bodies in hypertensive retinopathy and other diseases. Trans Ophthalmol Soc UK 1963;83:91–114.
23 Bayliss WM: On the local reactions of the arterial wall to changes of internal pressure. J Physiol 1902;28:220–231.
24 Pal J: Die Gefässkrisen. Leipzig, Hirzel, 1905.
25 Byrom FB: The caliber of the retinal arteries in hypertension. Am Heart J 1963;66:727–730.
26 Volhard F: Der arterielle Hochdruck. Ges innere Med, München 1923;35:134–184.
27 Wagener HP, Keith NM: Diffuse arteriolar disease with hypertension and the associated retinal lesions. Medicine (Baltimore) 1939;18:317–430.
28 Keith NM, Wagener HP, Barker NW: Some different types of essential hypertension: Their course and prognosis. Am J Med Sci 1939;197:332–343.
29 Wagener HP, Clay GE, Gipner JF: Classification of retinal lesions in the presence of vascular hypertension. Trans Am Ophthalmol Soc 1947;45:57–73.
30 Leishman R: The eye in general vascular disease – Hypertension and arteriosclerosis. Br J Ophthalmol 1957;41:641–701.
31 Mylius K: Funktionelle Veränderungen am Gefässsystem der Netzhaut. Abh Augenheilk 1928;10:1–82.
32 Wagener HP: Arterioles of retina in toxemia of pregnancy. JAMA 1933;101:1380–1384.
33 Wagener HP: Spasm and organic arterial lesions in the retina. Trans Am Acad Ophthalmol Otolaryngol 1958;62:357–393.
34 Juler FA: Some points in the operation for acute glaucoma. Trans Ophthalmol Soc UK 1949;69:3–15.
35 Dollery CT, Hill DW, Hodge JV: The response of normal retinal blood vessels to angiotensin and noradrenaline. J Physiol 1963;165:500–507.
36 Hill DW, Dollery CT: Calibre changes in retinal arterioles. Trans Ophthalmol Soc UK 1963;83:61–70.
37 Ramalho PS, Dollery CT: Hypertensive retinopathy: Calibre changes in retinal blood vessels following blood-pressure reduction and inhalation of oxygen. Circulation 1968;37:580–588.
38 Abt K, Brueckner R: Netzhautgefässspasmen bei artifiziell hypertonischen Ratten. Ophthalmologica 1950;119:17–43.
39 Robert A, Nezamis JE: Hypertensive eye lesions in the rat: Effect of carotid ligation. Experientia 1957;13:457–459.
40 Byrom FB: The nature of malignancy in hypertensive diseases. Evidence from the retina of the rat. Lancet 1963;i:516–520.
41 Engerman RL, Meyer RK, Buesseler JA: Effects of alloxan diabetes and steroid hypertension on retinal vasculature. Am J Ophthalmol 1964;58:965–978.
42 Uyama M: Ophthalmological studies on experimental hypertension. I. A clinical observation of the eye of the rat with experimental renal hypertension. Nippon Ganka Gakkai Zasshi 1966;70:132–149.
43 Bellhorn RW: Pathophysiology of retinal vessels in experimentally hypertensive rats; M Sc thesis, New York University, 1966.
44 Nakazawa T: Studies on the changes in the retinal vessels of the rat with experimental renal hypertension. Nippon Ganka Gakkai Zasshi 1969;73:417–432.
45 Kawaguchi H: A study on experimental hypertension. 1. Fundus findings and histopathologic findings of DCA-induced hypertensive rabbits. Nippon Ganka Gakkai Zasshi 1968;72:77–92.
46 Laughlin RC, Thomas CB, Friedenwald JS: The retinal arteries in experimental renal hypertension: The significance of localized caliber constriction. Bull Johns Hopk Hosp 1940;67:79–91.
47 Oka Y, Nomura T, Nakamura M, Okabayashi T: Ophthalmological studies on perinephritis hypertension in monkeys: Pathogenesis of retinal changes. Nippon Ganka Gakkai Zasshi 1975;79:904–914.
48 McMichael J: Reorientations in hypertensive disorders. Br Med J 1961;ii:1310–1314.
49 Stokoe NL: Fundus changes in hypertension. A long-term clinical study; in Cant JS (ed): The Ocular Circulation in Health and Disease. London, Kimpton, 1969, pp 117–135.
50 Michaelson IC, Eliakim M, Avshalom A, et al: An approach to the investigation of the vascular changes in the fundus of the eye in hypertension and arteriosclerosis. Acta XX Conc Ophthalm Germania 1966 I;1967:207–219.
51 Evelyn KA, Nicholls JVV, Turnbull W: A method of grading and recording. The retinal changes in essential hypertension. Am J Ophthalmol 1958;45:165–179.
52 Ashton N: The eye in malignant hypertension. Trans Am Acad Ophthalmol Otolaryngol 1972;76:17–40.
53 Reed RK, Sapirstein LA, Southard FD, et al: Effects of nembutal and yohimbine on chronic renal

hypertension in the rat. Am J Physiol 1944;141:707–712.
54 Green DM, Saunders FJ, Wahlgren N, et al: Self-sustaining post-DCA hypertensive cardiovascular disease. Am J Physiol 1952;170:94–106.
55 Brunson JG, Davis RL: Systemic fibrinoid diseases; similarity to experimental lesions in rabbits. Arch Pathol 1955;60:593–609.
56 Kincaid-Smith P: Malignant hypertension: mechanisms and management. Pharmacol Ther 1980; 9:245–269.
57 Giese J: The Pathogenesis of Hypertensive Vascular Disease. Copenhagen, Munkssgaard, 1966.
58 Carl T: Ein Beitrag zur pathologischen Anatomie des Auges bei Nierenleiden. Wiesbaden, Bergmann, 1887.
59 Buechner F: Die Rolle des Herzmuskels bei der Angina pectoris. Beitr Pathol Anat 1932;89:644–667.

Dr. S. S. Hayreh
Department of Opthalmology
University of Iowa
Hospitals and Clinics
Iowa City, IA 52242 (USA)

Ophthalmologica 1989;198:197–215

Cotton-Wool Spots (Inner Retinal Ischemic Spots) in Malignant Arterial Hypertension

Sohan Singh Hayreh, Gary E. Servais, Prem Singh Virdi

Department of Ophthalmology, University of Iowa, Iowa City, Iowa, USA

Key Words. Arterial hypertension · Blood pressure · Cotton-wool spots · Hypertensive retinopathy · Inner retinal ischemic spots · Malignant arterial hypertension · Retina · Retinal arteriolar occlusion · Retinal capillary obliteration · Soft exudates

Abstract. We produced experimental renovascular malignant arterial hypertension by modified Goldblatt's procedures, in 60 rhesus monkeys. Hypertensive retinopathy was studied in detail (by ophthalmoscopy, and stereoscopic color fundus photography and fluorescein fundus angiography on long-term follow-up). Cotton-wool spots (CWSs) were found to be an important, early retinal lesion. On ophthalmoscopy, they had a characteristic appearance. Fluorescein fundus angiography of these lesions revealed focal retinal capillary nonperfusion. The CWSs usually lasted for over 3 weeks and resolved within 6 weeks, leaving permanent obliteration of the retinal capillaries in their distribution, secondary intraretinal microvascular abnormalities, and retinal nerve fiber loss. We discuss pathogenesis and other features of CWSs. There is overwhelming evidence that CWSs are due to occlusion of the terminal retinal arterioles, resulting in acute focal inner retinal ischemia; hence the scientifically valid term for them would be '*inner retinal ischemic spots*'.

Ever since the first clinical description of fundus changes in malignant hypertension in 1859 [1], cotton-wool spots (CWSs) have been emphasized as an important classical feature of hypertensive retinopathy in malignant arterial hypertension. In spite of the accumulation of an extensive literature on the subject, many aspects of these lesions, particularly their pathogenesis and fluorescein fundus angiographic pattern, still remain debatable. Many authors have concluded that CWSs are minute infarcts related to occlusion or spasm in retinal arterioles [2–5]. McLeod et al. [6], however, concluded that 'cotton-wool spots are not 'microinfarcts' of the inner retina, as defined hitherto'; similarly Hodge and Dollery [7] claimed to have found no positive evidence of vascular occlusion in these lesions. Likewise, the fluorescein fundus angiographic pattern of CWSs has been controversial, particularly the occurrence and mechanism of retinal capillary obliteration and fluorescein leakage. In the light of our studies and the evidence in the literature, we shall describe the clinical, ophthalmoscopic and fluorescein fundus angiographic patterns of CWSs in hypertensive retinopathy, and discuss their pathogenesis in detail.

Materials and Methods

In 60 adult, healthy rhesus monkeys we produced renovascular systemic malignant arterial hypertension. This was done by clamping the left renal artery by a modified Goldblatt's procedure, described in detail in another publication [8]. Two types of hypertensive experimental models were produced: a *one-kidney, one-clip* model (in 25 monkeys), and a *two-kidney, one-clip model* (in 35 monkeys). In the former, the normal right kidney was removed at the time when the left renal artery was clamped so that the animal was left with only one, ischemic kidney. In the two-kidney model, the animal had a normal right kidney and an ischemic left kidney.

In all the animals, we recorded blood pressure (BP) and fundus changes before renal artery clamping and serially thereafter. The BP was recorded by the auscultatory method, using a Doppler stethoscope and an infant arm cuff; details of this method are described elsewhere [8]. We could reliably record only the systolic BP. The fundus changes were recorded by direct and indirect ophthalmoscopy, and stereoscopic color fundus photography and fluorescein fundus angiography. In addition to these investigations, we also performed preoperative and postoperative renal function tests (blood urea and creatinine levels) and hematologic studies. The frequency of all these investigations depended on the severity of arterial hypertension and fundus lesions in each animal, and its general state of health, because fundus photography and fluorescein fundus angiography and the repeated nembutal anesthesia required for these procedures are highly stressful for sick, hypertensive animals; thus the follow-up for each animal was individualized to obtain the best possible information without risk to the animal's long-term survival.

For data analysis, in each monkey, we critically evaluated the record of BP, and the findings of ophthalmoscopy, and stereoscopic color fundus photography and fluorescein fundus angiography on CWSs and other fundus lesions during the longitudinal follow-up period. The data for each animal for the various fundus lesions were tabulated for the several parameters evaluated in this study, including BP, time since renal artery clamping, different ophthalmoscopic and fluorescein fundus angiographic features of each lesion, etc., separately for the one-kidney and two-kidney models. The data were finally collated and analyzed separately for the two models. The median (the 50th percentage point in data) and interquartile range (IQR; the difference between the 75th and 25th percentage points) are presented for most of the parameters because these statistics present a better picture of the center and spread of a distribution than do the mean and standard deviation when there are extreme values in the data, as was usually the case in this study. The Wilcoxon rank sum test and Spearman correlation coefficient were used to determine statistical significances.

Results

BP, Hypertensive Retinopathy and Follow-Up Period

Table 1 summarizes the data on the BP, incidence of hypertensive retinopathy and length of follow-up. The general BP changes in

Table 1. Length of follow-up, BP findings and hypertensive retinopathy in one-kidney and two-kidney animals

	One-kidney group (25 monkeys)			Two-kidney group (35 monkeys)		
	range	median	IQR	range	median	IQR
Follow-up period, months	1.2–57.3[1]	9.6[1]	19.2[1]	0.7–42.3	26.4	10.5
Time interval (days) from renal artery clamping to						
Onset of hypertension	2– 43	7	3	2–115	15	18
Maximum BP recorded	2–980	110	287	8–899	124	237
Onset of hypertensive retinopathy	12– 63[2]	22[2]	17[2]	8–302[3]	64[3]	44[3]
Highest BP recorded						
BP level, in mm Hg	178–260	220	30	160–260	204	50
% Rise from baseline BP	148–245	193	46	133–237	175	26
BP at onset of hypertensive retinopathy, mm Hg	164–225[2]	190[2]	21[2]	160–210[3]	178[3]	26[3]

1 In 20 animals that survived ≥3 weeks.
2 Hypertensive retinopathy seen in 19 one-kidney monkeys.
3 Hypertensive retinopathy seen in 19 two-kidney monkeys.

this experimental study are discussed elsewhere [8]. In our experience of dealing with over a hundred normal adult rhesus monkeys, we have found their normal median systolic BP to be 120 (IQR 15) mm Hg. Judging from BP levels seen in human arterial hypertension, we decided to consider a systolic BP of ≥160 mm Hg as hypertensive. Renovascular hypertension developed in all the 60 monkeys. It developed significantly ($p = 0.01$) earlier in the one-kidney than in the two-kidney model. One-kidney monkeys developed much more rapid and more severe hypertension than the two-kidney animals; however, there was no significant difference between the two models of hypertension in the one-time highest recorded BP (either in the time it took for the BP to reach the highest level or in the level of BP recorded [8]. Five of the 25 one-kidney monkeys died within 3 weeks after renal artery clamping, from complications of accelerated hypertension or uremia. Some evidence of hypertensive retinopathy developed in 19 one-kidney monkeys (out of the 20 surviving 3≥ weeks) and 19 of the 35 two-kidney monkeys.

Cotton-Wool Spots

CWSs developed in 17 one-kidney animals, involving both eyes in all, although initially they were seen in only one eye of 6 animals. CWSs were seen in 13 of the two-kidney animals.

a

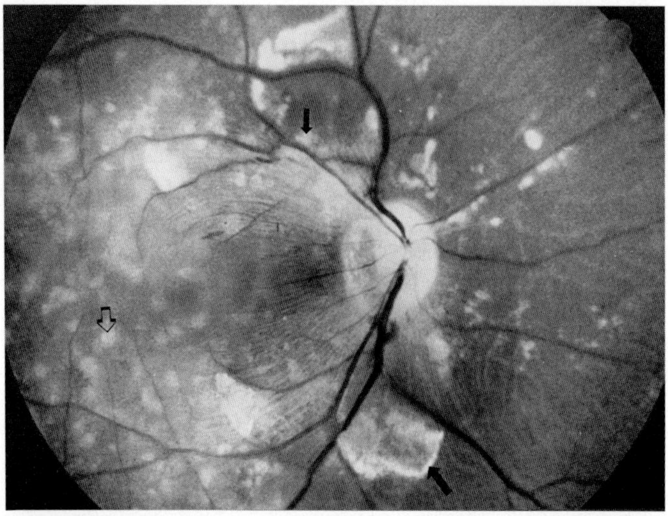

b

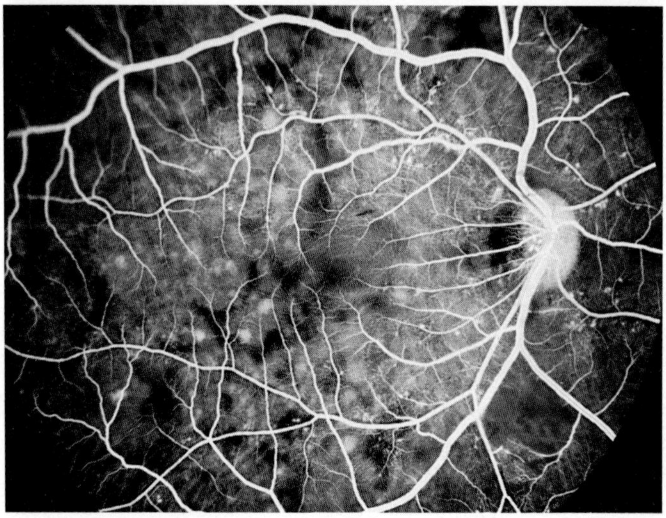

Fig. 1. Ophthalmoscopic (**a**) and fluorescein fundus angiographic (**b, c**) appearance in right eye of a one-kidney model monkey, 56 days after surgery with BP 238 mm Hg. **a** Multiple (CWSs (large arrow), FIPTs (small arrow) and acute focal retinal pigment epithelial lesions (hollow arrow), macular edema and macular serous retinal detachment. **b** Angiogram during retinal arteriovenous phase shows retinal capillary nonperfusion in the regions of the various CWSs, characteristic pin-point fluorescent spots in relation to the retinal arterioles and their branches in the distribution of the FIPTs, and subretinal fluorescent spots in the macular region due to acute focal retinal pigment epithelial lesions.

When the CWSs Appeared for the First Time. In the *one-kidney monkeys,* these developed 19–203 (median 49.5, IQR 35) days after the renal artery clamping, with a BP of 178–240 (median 199, IQR 25) mm Hg, and there was no statistically significant correlation between these two parameters. In the *two-kidney monkeys,* they appeared in 42–301 (median 87, IQR 36) days (except in 1 animal which did not develop noteworthy arterial hypertension for 2.5 years, and first developed CWSs in about 3 years), with a BP of 160–220 (median 187, IQR 30) mm Hg. The CWSs were almost invariably located in the distribution of the radial peripapillary capillaries (fig. 1–4) and there were additional CWSs in the peripapillary retina in

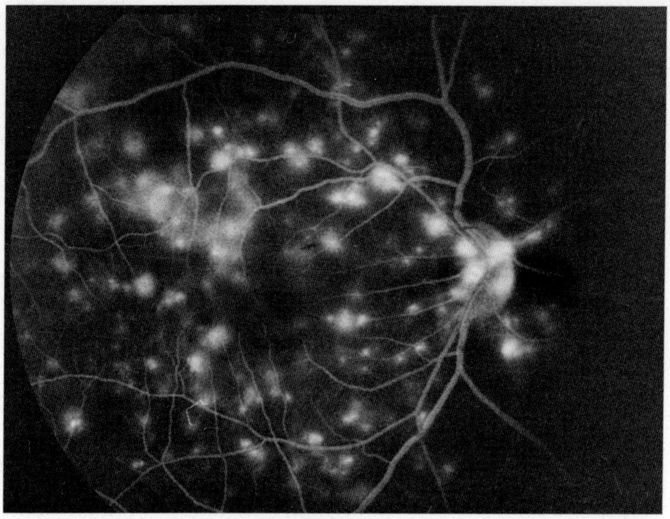

c

Fig. 1c. During the late phase of the angiography, there is characteristic fluorescein leakage from the FIPTs and the retinal pigment epithelial lesions, with no leakage in the distribution of the CWSs. Published courtesy of *Ophthalmology* 1986;93: 60–73 [9].

one third of the animals, but rarely elsewhere. At that stage, the number of CWSs tended to correspond with the severity of retinopathy in about half of the animals, but not in the other half. Rarely, CWSs were the first manifestation of hypertensive retinopathy.

When the CWSs Were Most Marked in an Animal. At this stage, the number of CWSs varied widely. In the *one-kidney model,* there were only one or two spots in 4, a moderate number in 9, and numerous (about 10 or more) in 4. At this phase, in 13 of the animals the severity of CWSs was significantly ($p<0.0001$) related to the overall severity of the retinopathy. CWSs were almost always located in the distribution of radial peripapillary capillaries (mostly along the temporal arcade of retinal vessels) and in about one half also in the peripapillary retina, and only rarely away from the temporal arcade of vessels or in the macular region. The BP at this stage was 162–240 (median 198, IQR 24) mm Hg, and the severity of CWSs at this stage showed no statistically significant correlation to the height of BP. In the *two-kidney model,* the maximum severity of CWSs seen in an animal, at its peak, was mild in 3 animals, moderate in 5 and extensive in 5.

Shape and Size of the CWSs. These were highly variable, depending upon the size of the arteriole involved and the area supplied by it (fig. 1a, 2a, 3a, 4a). In 1 animal a small arteriolar occlusion produced a big patch of retinal infarct superonasal to the fovea and this resembled a CWS in all aspects, including the capillary nonperfusion on fluorescein fundus angiography. The color, size and shape of the lesion were greatly influenced by the age of the CWSs – initially fluffy white lesions, they later changed to dull dry crumbling white material, shrinking in size, and finally disappearing.

Fluorescein Fundus Angiographic Findings. During the initial stages soon after the onset of CWSs: at this stage, during the very early phase of transit of the dye, retinal capillaries were not seen focally in the spots; this was essentially due to nonperfusion of the capillaries in the region of the CWSs (fig. 1b, 2b), but it is pos-

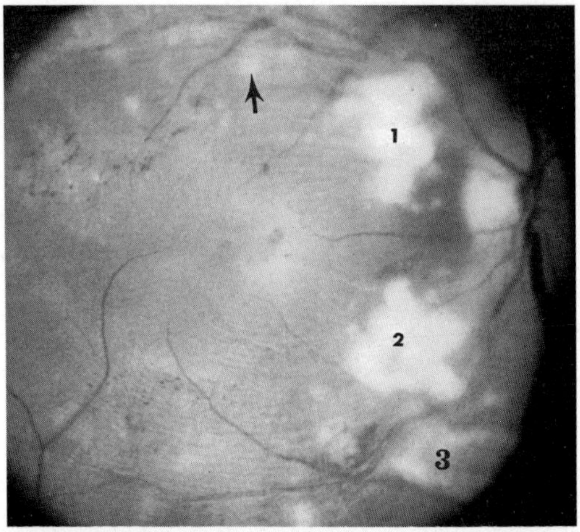

2a

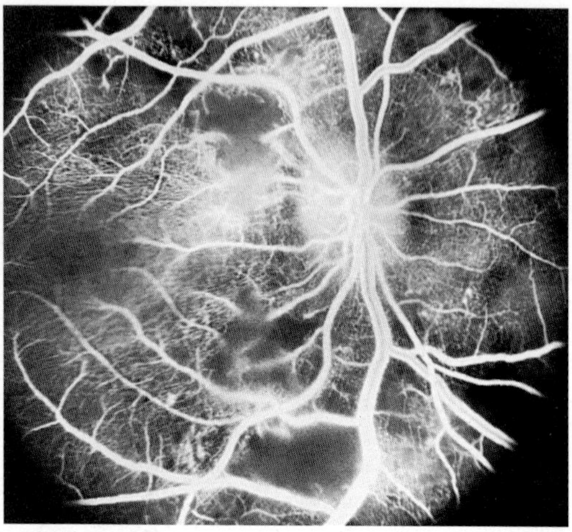
2b

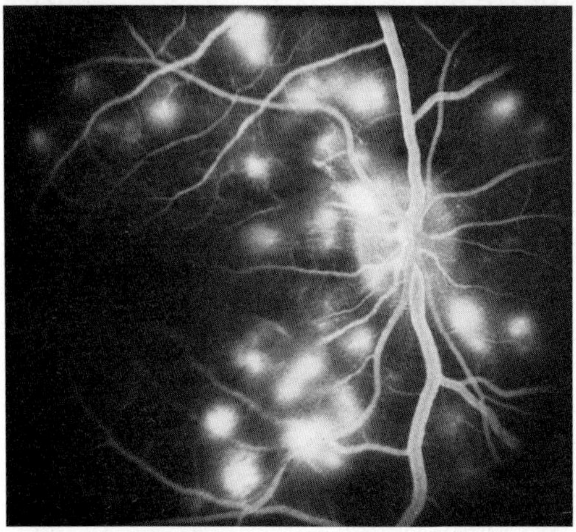
2c

Fig. 2. Ophthalmoscopic (**a**) and fluorescein angiographic (**b, c**) appearance in right eye of one-kidney monkey (day 56; BP 240 mm Hg). **a** Two fresh CWSs (No. 1 and 2), in addition to resolving CWS (No. 3) and FIPTs (arrow), marked macular edema and macular serous retinal detachment with opaque exudative subretinal fluid. **b** Angiogram during the retinal arteriovenous phase shows retinal capillary nonperfusion in the distribution of the fresh and resolving CWSs. **c** During the late phase of the angiography fluorescein leaking spots are seen only in the distribution of the FIPTs, and *none* in the region of the CWSs. In the region of the CWS No. 2, situated inferotemporal to the optic disk, there are some underlying FIPTs (best seen on stereoscopic examination) which are responsible for the fluorescein leakage in that area.

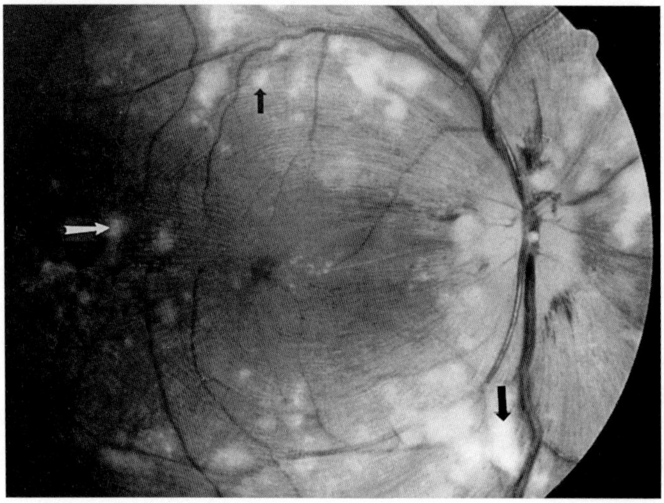
a

Fig. 3. Ophthalmoscopic appearance in right eye of a two-kidney monkey. **a** Fundus photograph (day 57; BP 190 mm Hg) shows multiple CWSs (large arrow), FIPTs (small arrow) and acute focal retinal pigment epithelial lesions (white arrow), and macular edema. Published courtesy of *Ophthalmology* 1986;93:74–87 [10].

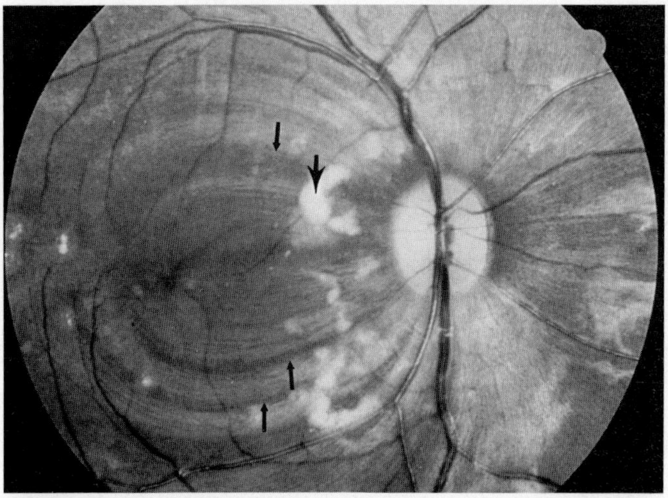

b

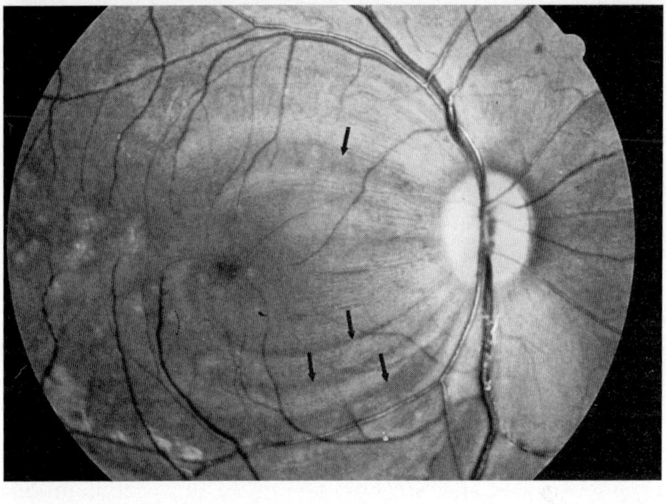

c

Fig. 3. b Fundus photograph (day 120) shows that the old CWSs have resolved and new ones have appeared (large arrow), with development of multiple areas of nerve fiber loss (seen as dark semicircular bands in the macular region; small arrows). **c** Fundus photograph (day 311) shows all CWSs have resolved, leaving multiple areas of nerve fiber bundle loss (arrows). Note also the presence of multiple focal retinal pigment epithelial lesions in the temporal part of the macular region.

sible that it could have been partly due to masking by the overlying opaque retina. During the later stages of the transit of the dye, most of the CWSs showed slow, delayed filling of the retinal capillaries from the adjacent capillaries.

During the terminal stages of CWSs: permanent retinal capillary obliteration was usually recorded about 5 weeks or more after the onset of CWSs, and from then on capillary obliteration progressed with time, so that prominent focal or extensive capillary obliteration was seen later in those areas (fig. 4b–6). The extent of retinal capillary obliteration in an eye depended essentially upon the extent and distribution of the CWSs. The capillary obliteration was almost always located in the distribution of radial peripapillary capillaries and the

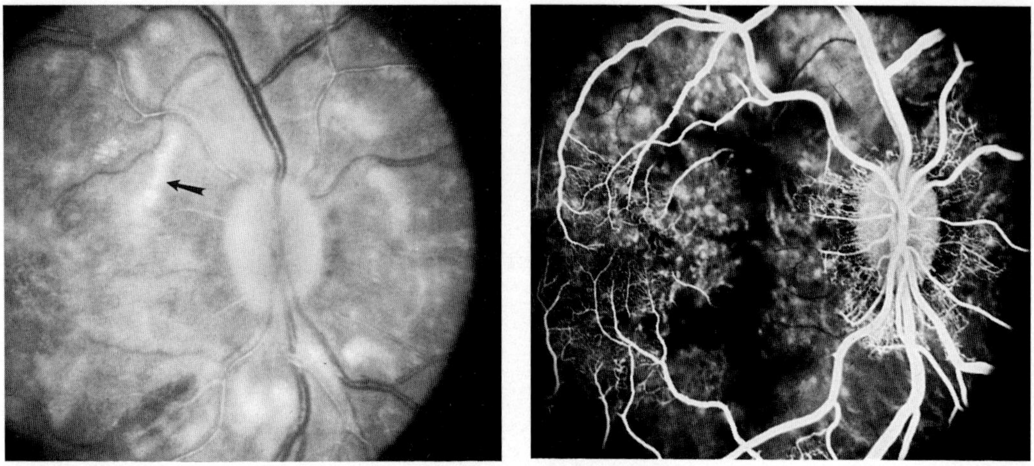

Fig. 4. Ophthalmoscopic (**a**) and fluorescein angiographic (**b**) appearance of right eye of a one-kidney monkey (day 131; BP 196 mm Hg). **a** Fundus photograph shows multiple active CWSs (arrow), retinal arteriolar sclerosis, and mild macular edema with flat macular serous retinal detachment. **b** Angiogram during the late retinal arteriovenous phase shows extensive retinal capillary nonperfusion in the distribution of the current and old CWSs.

peripapillary retina. The terminal retinal arteriole, corresponding to the distribution of a large patch of capillary obliteration, was occluded (fig. 4b, 5c, 6b) and frequently developed sheathing (usually from its origin from the main arcuate arteriole; fig. 4a, 6a). The sheathed retinal vessels were found to be completely occluded (fig. 4b, 6b). Stumps of the occluded arterioles were seen with focal capillary nonperfusion in their distribution. In addition, some eyes also showed variable reduction in the population of the retinal capillaries in the posterior pole as a whole (fig. 4–6). Retinal capillary obliteration was also responsible for the development of the secondary intraretinal microvascular abnormalities, described below.

CWSs in general showed no late staining on fluorescein fundus angiography (fig. 1, 2). In some eyes there was overlap between the CWSs and the focal intraretinal periarteriolar transudates [9] (FIPTs), and the late staining of the latter gave an erroneous impression of staining of the CWSs (fig. 1, 2). Very rarely, a resolving CWS showed some fluorescein leak. Intraretinal microvascular abnormalities (occasionally seen secondary to retinal capillary obliteration) showed late fluorescein staining (fig. 5). Some of the big retinal arterioles and venules passing through CWSs showed localized fluorescein leakage, as if focal ischemia had produced breakdown in the blood-retinal barrier in the large retinal vessels.

Life Cycle of CWSs. The CWSs took weeks to resolve. Some lasted longer than others, but usually it was more than 3 weeks and less than 6 (fig. 3). Since the fundus was not examined very frequently because of the dangers of anesthesia [8], it is not possible to give the exact duration of the CWSs. As the old spots resolv-

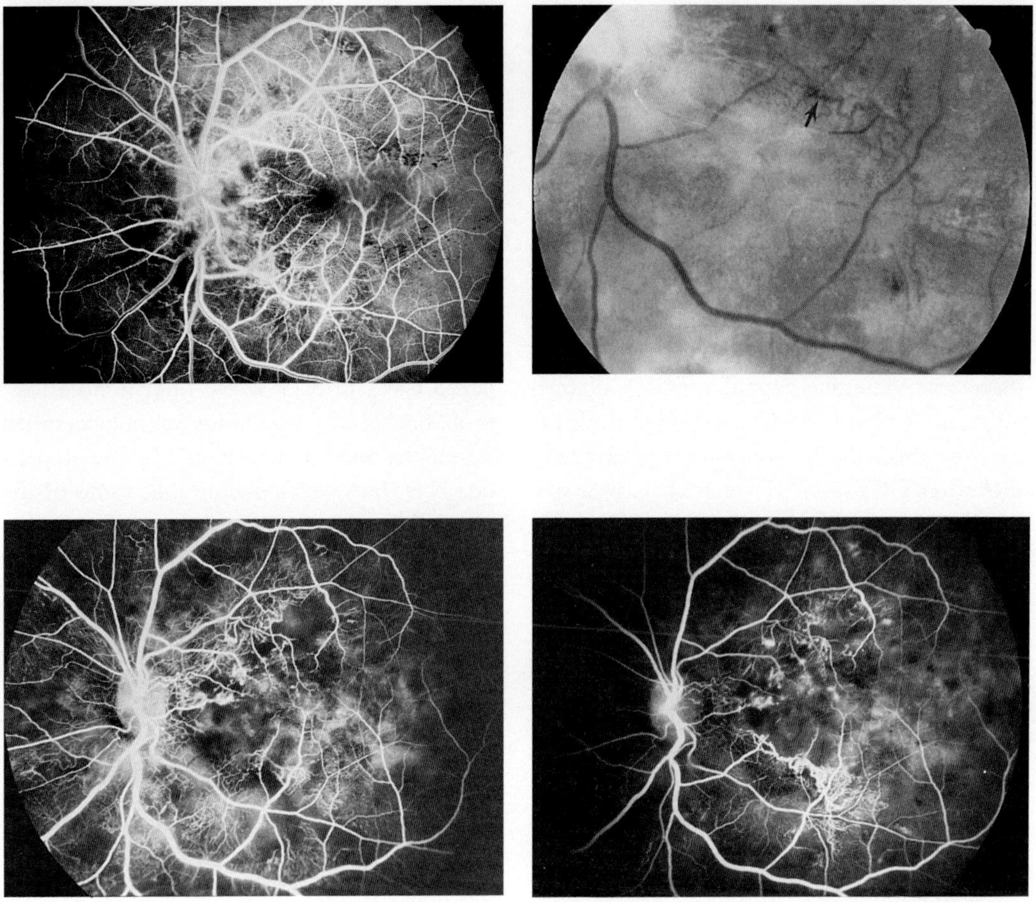

Fig. 5. Ophthalmoscopic (**b**) and fluorescein angiographic (**a, c–e**) appearance of left eye of a one-kidney monkey. **a** Angiogram (day 42; BP 200 mm Hg) shows almost normal retinal capillary filling during the retinal arteriovenous phase. Published courtesy of *Opthalmology* 1986;93:60–73 [9]. **b** Fundus photograph (day 120; BP of ≥200 mm Hg for about 3 months) shows intraretinal microvascular abnormalities (arrow) in the lower part of the macular region and retinal arteriolar sclerosis. Fluorescein angiography on that day, during retinal late arteriovenous (**c**), postvenous (**d**) and late phases (**e**) shows extensive retinal capillary nonperfusion in the macular region, marked reduction in the population of retinal capillaries elsewhere, and intraretinal microvascular abnormalities; compare the retinal capillary pattern in **a** with that in **c**.

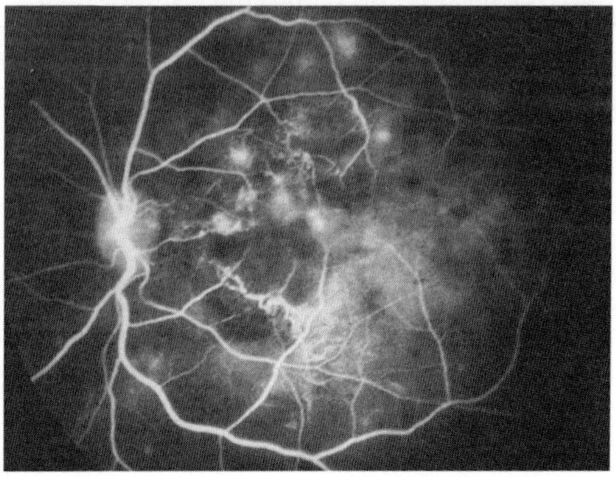

ed, new ones appeared from time to time (fig. 3) – in some one-kidney animals even up to about 10 months after the renal artery clamping. In the two-kidney model, the same sequence happened, but sometimes there were intervals when no CWSs were to be seen. In the two-kidney model, the CWSs kept appearing for 35 days to over 2 years (median 120 days, IQR 62), and when they resolved completely the BP was 130–250 (median 184, IQR 36) mm Hg. In the one-kidney model, once there was extensive retinal capillary obliteration, no further CWSs developed in those areas. Although the BP was almost always very high when CWSs were developing in these one kidney animals, we could not prove any definite correlation between the extent of CWSs and the height of BP. Nor was there any definite relationship in the two-kidney model animals between the height of the BP and the severity of CWSs, because in some of the animals, in spite of very high BP (as much as 220–250 mm Hg) either no CWSs developed or they resolved completely; yet in others with only minor hypertension, CWSs did develop.

Retinal Nerve Fiber Loss

As the CWSs resolved, nerve fiber loss in the retinal nerve fiber layer started to develop, its location depending upon the distribution of the CWSs (fig. 3). Definite nerve fiber bundle loss of variable degree was detected ophthalmoscopically in 12 of the 17 one-kidney animals with CWSs; in the remaining 5 most probably the loss of nerve fibers was more diffuse than localized, and ophthalmoscopically not apparent. The loss of nerve fibers was seen in 9 two-kidney animals – all these eyes had CWSs; in 4 animals of this group, with CWSs, no apparent nerve fiber loss could be detected – presumably the loss was too subtle to be detected ophthalmoscopically. The time interval between the onset of CWSs and that of nerve fiber loss could not be estimated accurately because of the gradual nature of the loss of nerve fibers and the time lapse between fundus examinations (for reasons mentioned above).

The loss of nerve fiber bundles was seen most commonly in the temporal arcuate distribution around the optic disk, i.e. in the distribution of the CWSs (fig. 3). There was usually a progressive increase in nerve fiber loss. In some eyes it was not always possible to correlate a CWS to each nerve fiber bundle loss, probably because the fundus was not examined frequently enough through the follow-up period. It is, however, possible that some of the nerve fiber loss could be due to hypertensive optic neuropathy [10].

Intraretinal Microvascular Abnormalities Associated with CWSs

There were almost always secondary to retinal capillary obliteration associated with CWSs. One or another of these abnormalities was seen in 8 one-kidney animals, but it was rare in the two-kidney monkeys because of their mild hypertensive retinopathy. Most of the abnormalities could be classified as follows:

Shunts Around the Areas with Capillary Obliteration (fig. 5). Some of these stained with fluorescein on angiography.

Stumps of the Occluded Capillaries. These were seen at the peripheral parts of the areas with capillary obliteration (fig. 2b, 4b, 5c). They leaked fluorescein, giving an impression of being microaneurysms.

Looped Convoluted Vessels. These were slightly larger than the retinal capillaries and leaked fluorescein during the late phase of fluorescein fundus angiography, producing a fluorescent spot the size of the looped vessel (fig. 5c–e). These fluorescent spots resembled

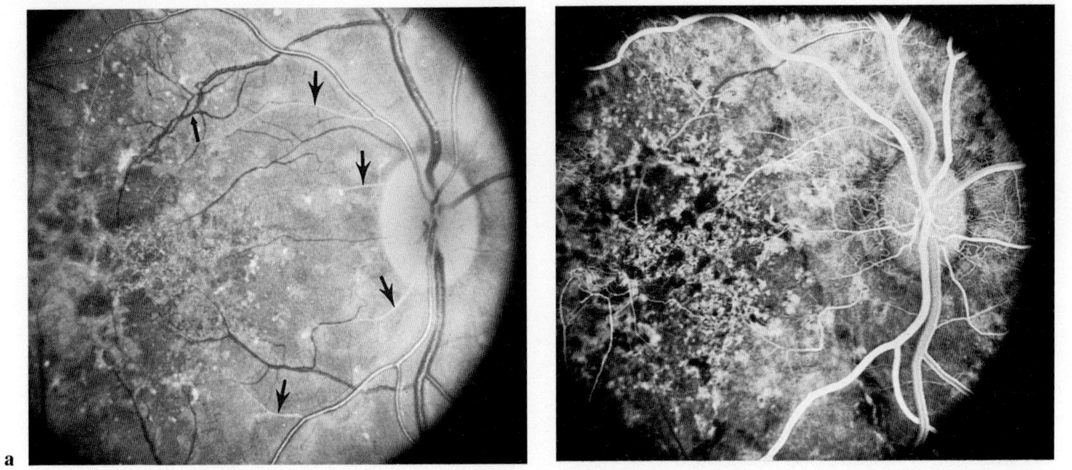

Fig. 6. Ophthalmoscopic (**a**) and fluorescein angiographic (**b**) appearance of left eye of a one-kidney monkey (day 403; BP 218 mm Hg). **a** Fundus photograph shows extensive late retinal pigment epithelial degenerative changes, retinal arteriolar sclerosis, sheathing of some of the retinal arterioles (large arrows), intraretinal microvascular abnormalities (small arrow) and optic atrophy. **b** Angiogram during the retinal arteriovenous phase, shows extensive retinal capillary nonperfusion, complete obliteration of the sheathed retinal arterioles, and extensive retinal pigment epithelial degenerative changes in the macular region.

those seen with FIPTs [9]. When these abnormalities showed leakage of fluorescein, the retina in that location was somewhat opaque on ophthalmoscopy, again mimicking FIPTs [9].

Comment

CWSs are seen in a variety of systemic thromboembolic disorders and constitute an important feature of hypertensive retinopathy. According to Leishman [4], CWSs are a feature of severe and fulminating hypertension, with diastolic BP 130 mm Hg or more. In the present study, the CWSs appeared when the median systolic BP was 199 mm Hg in the one-kidney model and 187 mm Hg in the two-kidney model. The hypertension developed significantly ($p = 0.01$) faster in the one-kidney model than in the two-kidney model [8], and the CWSs were seen in 85% of the one-kidney animals 49.5 days (median) after the renal artery clamping, but in only 37% of the two-kidney animals at 87 days (median). This indicates that the more accelerated the arterial hypertension, the higher the incidence of CWSs, and the earlier they develop.

Clinical Features of CWSs

Typically, CWSs are fluffy white focal areas of retinal opacity, having irregular polymorphous shapes, frequently with somewhat feathery margins (fig. 1a, 2a, 3a, b, 4a). They are located mostly in the nerve fiber layer on the retina, usually in the posterior pole (within a few disk diameters from the disk), essentially in the distribution of the radial peripapillary capillaries [11], and more closely related to the arterioles than to the venules. During the acute phase, they usually bulge slightly forward on the surface of the retina. The characteristic life cycle of a CWS is that it starts as a gray film, expands as a white creamy fluffy cloud and resolves into a dull fragmenting white patch before disappearing [7]. Finally, on complete resolution, it leaves a normal-looking transparent retina on ophthalmoscopy although fluorescein fundus angiography reveals permanent capillary nonperfusion on its location (fig. 4–6).

Differentiating Features between CWSs and the FIPTs

In the past, FIPTs (a retinal lesion recently discovered by us [9] and CWSs in malignant hypertension have mistakenly been considered one entity, because of the superficial ophthalmoscopic resemblance between the two lesions; this resulted in controversy on the fluorescein fundus angiographic pattern and pathogenesis of CWSs. FIPTs and CWSs are actually two distinct retinal lesions of malignant hypertension, differing very much in their ophthalmoscopic, fluorescein fundus angioraphic, life cycle and resolution patterns, and pathogeneses [9]. It is important that these two be differentiated from one another (fig. 1, 2]; the subject has been discussed by us in detail previously [9]; a brief summary is as follows:

Location in the Retina. CWSs are located in the superficial nerve fiber layer of the retina, whereas FIPTs are located in the deeper retinal layers. While CWSs are mostly located in the distribution of the radial peripapillary capillaries, FIPTs are invariably and typically located beside the major retinal arterioles and their main branches posteriorly.

Ophthalmoscopic Features. In contrast to the ophthalmoscopic features of CWSs described above, FIPTs are round or oval in shape, pinpoint to about a quarter of the disk diameter in size, and dull-white in color.

Fluorescein Angiographic Features. CWSs typically show retinal capillary nonperfusion in their location, progressively becoming more marked, with no corresponding fluorescein leakage. By contrast, FIPTs do not show any retinal capillary nonperfusion at any stage but show dilatation of precapillary terminal retinal arterioles in the deeper layers of the retina with focal leaking spots corresponding to the dilated arterioles, with the leaking spots appearing by the late arteriovenous phase, progressively increasing in size during the late phase, and located in the deeper retina.

Life Cycle and Resolution Pattern. CWSs last for 3–6 weeks and leave permanent focal retinal capillary non-perfusion areas and loss of retinal nerve fibers corresponding to the location of the CWSs. FIPTs, however, last for 2–3 weeks and resolve completely without leaving any permanent ophthalmoscopic, microvascular or fluorescein angiographic abnormality or any other detectable retinal abnormality. Grades of severity of CWSs and FIPTs were significantly different ($p<0.005$) in the present study, further indicating that the two lesions do not represent two stages in the same pathologic process. Also we never found any progression of FIPTs to CWSs, disproving the hypothesis of Dollery and coworkers [7, 12–16] that the two lesions represent a continuum with FIPTs as precursors of CWSs and that FIPTs are 'of aetiological importance in the causation of the cotton-wool spots' [7, 15] (hence they included both the lesions under the description of 'soft exudates').

Pathogenesis. All the available evidence indicates that the CWS is an acute focal retinal ischemic lesion, mainly involving the surface nerve fiber layer in the region of the radial peripapillary capillaries. By contrast, the FIPT is an exudative retinal lesion, caused by breakdown of the blood-retinal barrier in precapillary retinal arterioles in the deeper layers of the retina, due to dilatation of the arterioles from failure of autoregulation secondary to an accelerated rise of BP.

Fluorescein Fundus Angiographic Findings of 'Soft Exudates' in Malignant Arterial Hypertension Described by Dollery and Coworkers [7, 12–16]

These authors were the first to conduct fluorescein fundus angiographic studies in malignant hypertension in man and monkeys. Their studies formed the basis of our understanding of the angiographic findings in CWSs as well as other lesions in hypertensive retinopathy. According to them, in CWSs seen with hypertensive retinopathy, there were circumferential microaneurysms, central capillary closure, and fluorescein leaks from the region with microaneurysms. They found microaneurysms, dilated capillaries and tortuous small venules in 84% of the 'soft exudates' seen in patients. They reported restoration of capillary filling in many of the 'soft exudates' and felt that this reversible obstruction of the capillaries was probably due to shielding of the fluorescence by the opacity of the 'soft exudate'. They further added that there were often localized diffuse leaking points on or near feeding arterioles (not necessarily within the area enclosed by the 'soft exudates'), that some 'soft exudates' do not fluoresce and that, rarely, capillary closure may persist after resolution of the 'soft exudates'. However, Dollery and coworkers [7, 12–16] were unaware of the existence of FIPTs and therefore considered both FIPTs and CWSs as 'soft exudates', in all their studies. This misunderstanding makes it hard to evaluate their interpretation and findings on CWSs.

Gass [17] also reported the presence of dilated capillaries and microaneurysms, often arranged in a wreath-like fashion around the areas of poor capillary perfusion, patchy leakage of dye, typically in areas showing capillary dilatation, and sometimes diffusion of the dye into areas of poor capillary perfusion. According to him, angiographic and histopathologic findings suggest that focal areas of capillary ischemia and surrounding capillary changes may persist after clearing of CWSs, and that reversal of severe alterations in the capillary bed was unlikely. This contradicts the claim of Hodge and Dollery [7] that angiographic findings resolve completely in some patients after successful treatment of hypertension.

The fluorescein fundus angiographic findings of the present study are described in detail above. There was evidence of occlusion of terminal retinal arterioles and nonperfusion of the retinal capillaries in the area of the CWSs, with permanent capillary nonperfusion seen from about 5 weeks after the onset of CWSs, and from then on capillary obliteration was a progressive process (Fig. 1, 2, 4–6). The retinal capillary obliteration produced secondary intraretinal microvascular abnormalities, including shunts around the areas of capillary obliteration, microaneurysms, and looped convoluted vessels (fig. 4b, 5c, d). The microaneurysms really represented stumps of the occluded capillaries and were not true microaneurysms. Fluorescein leaked from the microaneurysms, shunts around the areas of capillary nonperfusion, and looped vessels; during the acute phase, however, the CWSs in general showed no fluorescein leakage or staining (fig. 1, 2). We feel the fluorescein leakage during the acute phase of the 'soft exudates' reported by Dollery and coworkers [7, 12–16] in fact represented leakage from FIPTs, and not from CWSs (fig. 1, 2). In our study, these two lesions sometimes overlaid one another, so that the fluorescein leakage from the FIPTs could well be attributed to the CWSs [9].

The life span of CWSs has been described as 4–6 weeks [4, 13] and 6–12 weeks [7] in man and 7–14 days in pigs [18]. In the present study, the CWSs usually lasted for 3 weeks and resolved within 6 weeks – some faster than others.

Pathologic Findings

'Cytoid bodies' were first described by Heymann [19] in 1856 in a case of Bright's disease and he regarded them as degenerate ganglion cells. But Müller [20], in 1858, showed that they were swollen varicose nerve fibers. Since then a large literature has accumulated on the subject, indicating that CWSs are focal areas of axonal swelling [5, 20–23]. Electron microscopy has confirmed that cytoid bodies are distended endings of disrupted nerve axons [5, 24–26]. In experimental CWSs, axoplasmic flow studies have revealed that the axonal swelling and collection of cytoplasmic organelles on their peripheral border and on the border nearest to the optic disk are caused by obstruction of orthograde and retrograde axoplasmic flows respectively, by ischemia [6].

Pathogenesis

Since 1929 many authors have concluded that CWSs are minute infarcts, related to occlusion or spasm in retinal arterioles [2–4]. There is considerable clinical and experimental evidence to support that view. For example, CWSs have been produced by experimental occlusion of precapillary retinal arterioles [18, 27, 28] and are also common in many systemic thromboembolic disorders. In histopathological studies, Leishman [4] found the CWSs related to a small thrombotic arteriole; however, Ashton and Harry [5] did not find thrombotic arterioles but did find occluded arterioles. Ashton [29], in his India-ink-injected specimens, found no filling of the capillaries in the CWSs, and attributed that obliteration largely to swelling of the nerve fibers. However, later on, in trypsin digestion of the retina with CWSs, injected with India ink, Ashton and Harry [5] found the intact skeleton of the capillaries in the distribution of the CWSs, but the capillaries did not fill with the ink. In flat preparation of the retina, they found terminal or precapillary arterioles supplying the CWSs obstructed. The occluded arterioles and associated capillaries showed fatty changes, and loss of endothelial and pericyte nuclei. The fatty changes were first shown by Verwey [30] in 1927 and subsequently by a host of other authors. Thus, Ashton and Harry [5] concluded that CWSs in severe hypertension are a result of sudden occlusion of a small arteriole and that CWSs represent pale infarcts. They also commonly found vascular dilatation and microaneurysms at the margins of the CWSs and, according to them, it was unusual to see these vascular changes elsewhere in the retina in hypertension. The cause of terminal retinal arteriolar occlusion in malignant hypertension is still not clear, and is most probably fibrinoid necrosis (also called 'fibrinous vasculosis'), a basic pathologic lesion of malignant hypertension. In our experimental study (as well as clinical experience in patients with hypertensive retinopathy), there has been definite fluorescein fundus angiographic evidence of occlusion of terminal retinal arterioles and nonperfusion of the retinal capillaries in the area of the CWSs (fig. 1b, 2b, 4b, 5c, 6b), as well as retinal nerve fiber loss corresponding to the distribution and development of the CWSs (fig. 3).

In studies on experimental arterial hypertension, focal constriction of systemic vessels has been reported, e.g., in mesenteric [31, 32] and intracranial arteries [31, 33–36] of rats and cerebral arteries in monkeys [37]. In some of them, the spasm progressed to fibrinoid necrosis [31, 38]. Meyer et al. [36] stated that cerebral arteriolar constriction and spasm result from a circulating vasoconstrictor factor that renders the smooth muscle of the arteriolar wall of cerebral vessels increasingly irritable, so that they respond to a normal or raised intraluminal pressure by excessive constriction – an excess 'Bayliss effect' [39], and this can be counteracted by lowering BP. Since the arterioles in the territory of an occluded cerebral vessel constrict in severe hypertension, the collateral circulation is reduced and the territory supplied by an occluded vessel may be rendered more ischemic. Because retinal and cerebral vessels have many common anatomic and physiologic properties, the above findings in cerebral circulation may be applicable to the terminal retinal arterioles. Ashton and Harry [5] postulated that in the formation of the CWSs, the possible sequence of events was as follows: initial gradual narrowing of the retinal arteriole → cutting down of circulation → fatty degenerative changes in the endothelium of the capillaries supplied by it → disturbances in permeability → leakage of fluid into the surrounding cells. In the involved area of the retina this would consequently produce anoxic swelling of the neural tissue. Thus, they believed, a fall in the capillary pressure with rise in the tissue pressure → collapse of the capillaries → fatty degeneration. Adjacent or surrounding capillaries with normal circulation become dilated, irregular and many of them show microaneurysms.

McLeod et al. [6] thought that the opaque lesion of CWSs represented accumulated axoplasm and cytoplasmic debris in the nerve fiber layer due to obstruction of orthograde or retrograde axoplasmic transport, and not microinfarcts of the inner retina. Hodge and Dollery [7] reported that they failed to find on fluorescein fundus angiography or ophthalmoscopy any positive evidence of retinal vascular occlusion, and postulated that CWSs were due to functional obliteration of the retinal capillaries; this impression was most probably caused by the authors' misdiagnosis of FIPTs as CWSs in their study (as discussed above), since the former show neither arteriolar occlusion nor capillary obliteration [9]. Garner and coworkers [14, 15] and Ashton [40] investigated the pathogenesis of retinal fibrinous vasculosis in malignant hypertension and its role in the pathogenesis of CWSs. This was an excellent pathologic study on the subject, but, unfortunately, its results and their interpretation were, again, vitiated by lumping together CWSs and FIPTs as one lesion [7, 12, 13, 16] (Dollery and co-workers as collaborators in this study were responsible for the clinical and fluorescein fundus angiographic interpretation of these lesions); this clinical misunderstanding distorted their interpretation of the pathological findings and hence their hypothesis. Garner [personal commun. December 1987], in view of our recent discovery of FIPTs as separate lesions, quite different from CWSs [9], now believes that it is reasonable to speculate that spasm of the terminal retinal arterioles may lead to thrombosis in the arterioles which would then lead to permanent closure of the terminal retinal arterioles and focal nonperfusion of the retinal capillaries in the CWSs without any leakage.

CWSs are usually located in the distribution of the radial peripapillary capillaries of the retina. These capillaries, as compared to ordinary retinal capillaries, have some characteristic features [11], including the following: (1) They are long straight capillaries, measuring several hundred micrometers to several millimeters. (2) They form the most superficial layer, lying among the superficial nerve fibers near the optic disk, mainly in the area superotemporal and inferotemporal to the disk and to a lesser extent on the nasal side of the disk. (3) They rarely anastomose with each other. (4) They arise from peripapillary retinal arterioles lying deeper in the retina and drain into retinal venules or veins on the optic disk. These features of radial peripapillary capillaries, and the much thicker nerve fiber layer in their distribution, could explain the distribution of CWSs. However, we still do not know the exact reasons for the special vulnerability of these vessels in the development of CWSs.

Retinal Capillary Changes in Malignant Hypertension

Capillary obliteration is a hallmark of CWSs, and as such this is seen frequently in retinopathy with malignant hypertension. Apart from the occlusion of terminal retinal arterioles, other mechanisms for capillary obliteration have also been postulated; these include the following:

(1) Hodge and Dollery [7] postulated that leaking retinal vessels cause local accumulation of edema fluid and the expanding pool of fluid may compress and obliterate the underlying capillaries to produce CWSs. However, this is based on their conflation of FIPTs with CWSs (as discussed above). We find no basis for this speculation.

(2) It has been speculated that retinal capillary obliteration is the result of serofibrinous insudation into the wall of the capillaries, similar to that postulated for the terminal arterioles [14, 15, 40].

(3)Garner and associates [14, 15, 40] postulated that the endothelial cell damage was due to anoxia from closure of the terminal arteriole and not a direct effect of the hypertensive state. Ashton and Harry [5] put forward the view that capillaries distal to the point of fibrinoid necrosis (and consequent arteriolar obstruction) degenerate because they are not perfusing. Endothelial cell contraction has also been thought to be responsible for capillary closure [14, 15, 40]. It is possible that endothelial cell swelling contributes to the narrowing in some instances, although this lacks proof. The late onset of permanent capillary obliteration at the sites of CWSs seen in the present study may be due to ischemic damage to capillaries.

The retinal capillary obliteration in the present study produced secondary intraretinal microvascular abnormalities, including microaneurysms, shunts around the areas of capillary obliteration, looped convoluted vessels, venous collaterals and arteriovenous shunts (fig. 5c–e). The pathogenesis of microaneurysms in malignant hypertension is still unknown. The intact capillaries in the immediate neighborhood of the avascular area frequently develop microaneurysms [41, 42]. In malignant hypertension Wexler and Branower [41] found dilatation and sacculation of the some of arterial capillaries, and focal reduplication of the basement membrane at the point of its sacculation. These changes produce capillary lesions resembling microaneurysms, similar to the ones seen in diabetes. According to them, these capillary lesions represent a specific disturbance seen only in malignant hypertension and not in benign hypertension or hypertension due to other causes. In diabetes, the lesions are seen predominantly in the venous capillary system. Our studies indicated that microaneurysms seen at the margin of the avascular area of CWSs may simply represent stumps of the surviving and perfusing retinal capillaries.

Conclusions

Thus, there is overwhelming evidence in the literature and also in the present study that CWSs are due to occlusion of the terminal retinal arterioles, with focal nonperfusion of the retinal capillaries in their distribution, resulting in acute focal inner retinal ischemia. Our studies also indicate that permanent retinal capillary obliteration in the distribution of the CWSs is secondary to ischemia. This is because during the early life of the CWS, retinal capillaries in the distribution of the CWS filled slowly from the adjacent retinal capillaries, but 5 weeks or longer after the onset the involved retinal capillaries were permanently obliterated.

Terminology

We would like to clarify the current confusion on the correct terminology to denote this lesion, which has been called by several different names, e.g., pathologically 'cytoid bodies', and clinically 'soft exudates' and 'cotton-wool spots' (or patches) [4, 43]. The term 'soft exudate' is wrong since these are not exudates at all (as is evident from the discussion above) and there is absolutely no justification for it. 'Cotton-wool spot' simply describes the ophthalmoscopic appearance during the acute phase, without giving any information about pathogenesis or any other feature. Based on the available evidence on the pathogenesis and other features of this lesion, we recommend the use of term 'inner retinal ischemic spot' (IRIS for short) because this is a truly descriptive and pathogenetic term.

Acknowledgments

We are grateful to Dr. Robert F. Woolson and Dr. Marie R. Klugman of the Department of Preventive Medicine (Biostatistics) for their help with the statistical analyses of the data, to Mrs. Ellen Ballas and Mrs. Georgiane Parkes-Perret for their secretarial help, to Mr. James Swaner for the technical help, and to the Photography Department for the illustrations. This investigation was supported by a research grant from the National Eye Institute (EY-1576) and in part by an unrestricted grant from Research to Prevent Blindness, Inc., and from the Alcon Research Institute.

References

1 Liebreich R: Ophthalmoskopischer Befund bei Morbus Brightii. Graefes Arch Clin Exp Ophthalmol 1859;5:265–268.
2 Volhard F: Die Pathogenese der Retinitis albuminurica. Zentralbl Gesamte Ophthalmol 1929;20: 627–628.
3 Friedenwald JS: A new approach to some problems of retinal vascular disease. Am J Ophthalmol 1949;32:487–498.
4 Leishman R: The eye in general vascular disease – Hypertension and arteriosclerosis. Br J Ophthalmol 1957;41:641–701.
5 Ashton N, Harry H: The pathology of cotton-wool spots and cytoid bodies in hypertensive retinopathy and other diseases. Trans Ophthalmol Soc UK 1963;83:91–114.
6 McLeod D, Marshall J, Kohner EM, et al: The role of axoplasmic transport in the pathogenesis of retinal cotton-wool spots. Br J Ophthalmol 1977;61:177–191.
7 Hodge JV, Dollery CT: Retinal soft exudates. Q J Med 1964;117–131.
8 Hayreh SS, Servais GE, Virdi PS, et al: Fundus lesions in malignant hypertension. III. Arterial

blood pressure, biochemical and fundus changes. Ophthalmology 1986;93:45–59.
9 Hayreh SS, Servais GE, Virdi PS: Fundus lesions in malignant hypertension. IV. Focal intra-retinal periarteriolar transudates. Ophthalmology 1986;93:60–73.
10 Hayreh SS, Servais GE, Virdi PS: Fundus lesions in malignant hypertension. V. Hypertensive optic neuropathy. Ophthalmology 1986;93:74–87.
11 Henkind P: New observations on the radial peripapillary capillaries. Invest Ophthalmol 1967;6:103–108.
12 Dollery CT, Hodge JV, Engel M: Studies of the retinal circulation with fluorescein. Br Med J 1962;ii:1210–1215.
13 Dollery CT, Hodge JV: Hypertensive retinopathy studied with fluorescein. Trans Ophthalmol Soc UK 1963;83:115–126.
14 Garner A: Experimental Hypertensive Retinopathy; PhD thesis, London, 1972.
15 Garner A, Ashton N, Tripathy R, et al: Pathogenesis of hypertensive retinopathy: An experimental study in the monkey. Br J Ophthalmol 1975;59: 3–44.
16 Dollery CT: Microcirculatory changes and the cotton-wool spot. Proc R Soc Med 1969;62:1267–1269.
17 Gass JDM: A fluorescein angiographic study of macular dysfunction secondary to retinal vascular disease. III. Hypertensive retinopathy. Arch Ophthalmol 1968;80:569–582.
18 Dollery CT, Henkind P, Paterson JW, et al: Ophthalmoscopic and circulatory changes in focal retinal ischaemia. Br J Ophthalmol 1966;50:285–324.
19 Heymann FM: Über Amaurose bei Brightischer Krankheit, und Fettdegeneration der Netzhaut. Graefes Arch Clin Exp Ophthalmol 1856;2: 137–150.
20 Müller H: Anatomische Beiträge zur Ophthalmologie. Graefes Arch Clin Exp Ophthalmol 1858; 4:363–388.
21 Leber T: Die Krankheiten der Netzhaut; in Graefe-Saemisch: Handbuch der Gesamten Augenheilkunde, vol 7/2. Leipzig, Englemann, 1915, p 840.
22 Koyanagi Y: Die Bedeutung der Gefässkreuzung für die Entstehung der Astthrombose der retinalen Zentralvene. Klin Monatsbl Augenheilkd 1928; 81:219–231.
23 Wolter JR: Pathology of a cotton-wool spot. Am J Ophthalmol 1959;48:473–485.
24 Shakib M, Ashton N: Ultrastructural changes in focal retinal ischaemia. Br J Ophthalmol 1966;50:325–384.
25 Inomata H, Ikui H, Kimura K: Fine structure of cytoid bodies. Jap J Ophthalmol 1967;11:1–14.
26 Ashton N: Pathophysiology of retinal cotton-wool spots. Br Med Bull 1970;26:143–150.
27 Gay AJ, Goldor H, Smith M: Chorioretinal vascular occlusions with latex spheres. Invest Ophthalmol 1964;3:647–656.
28 Ashton N, Henkind P: Experimental occlusion of retinal arterioles (using graded glass ballotini). Br J Ophthalmol 1965;49:225–234.
29 Ashton N: Diabetic retinopathy. A new approach. Lancet 1959;ii:625–630.
30 Verwey BC de la F: Über die Arteriosklerose der Netzhaut und ihre Bedeutung für die Genese der Retinitis albuminurica. Klin Monatsbl Augenheilkd 1927;79:148–158.
31 Byrom FB: The pathogenesis of hypertensive encephalopathy and its relation to the malignant phase of hypertension. Experimental evidence from the hypertensive rat. Lancet 1954;ii:201–211.
32 Giese J: Acute hypertensive vascular disease I. Relation between blood pressure changes and vascular lesions in different forms of acute hypertension. Acta Path Microbiol Scand 1964;62:481–496.
33 Byrom FB: The calibre of the cerebral arteries in experimental hypertension. Proc R Soc Med 1968;61:605–606.
34 Byrom FB: The Hypertensive Vascular Crisis. An Experimental study. London, Heinemann, 1969.
35 Meyer JS, Waltz AG, Gotoh F: Pathogenesis of cerebral vasospasm in hypertensive encephalopathy. I. Effects of acute increases in intraluminal blood pressure on pial blood flow. Neurology 1960;10: 735–744.
36 Meyer JS, Waltz AG, Gotoh F: Pathogenesis of cerebral vasospasm in hypertensive encephalopathy. II. The nature of increased irritability of smooth muscle of pial arterioles in renal hypertension. Neurology 1960;10:859–867.
37 Rodda R, Denny-Brown D: The cerebral arterioles in experimental hypertension. I. The nature of arteriolar constriction and its effects on the collateral circulation. Am J Pathol 1966;49:53–76.
38 Rodda R, Denny-Brown D: The cerebral arterioles in experimental hypertension. II. The development of arteriolonecrosis. Am J Pathol 1966;49: 365–382.
39 Bayliss WM: On the local reactions of the arterial

wall to changes of internal pressure. J Physiol 1902;28:220–231.

40 Ashton N: The eye in malignant hypertension. Trans Am Acad Ophthalmol Otolaryngol 1972;76:17–40.

41 Wexler D, Branower G: Retinal capillary lesions in malignant hypertension. Arch Ophthalmol 1950;44:539–548.

42 Ashton N: Retinal micro-aneurysms in the non-diabetic subject. Br J Ophthalmol 1951;35:189–212.

43 Wagener HP, Clay GE, Gipner JF: Classification of retinal lesions in the presence of vascular hypertension. Trans Am Ophthalmol Soc 1947;45:57–73.

Dr. S. S. Hayreh
Department of Ophthalmology
The University of Iowa Hospitals and Clinics
Iowa City, IA 52242 (USA)

Ophthalmologica 1989;198:216–229

Retinal Lipid Deposits in Malignant Arterial Hypertension

Sohan Singh Hayreh, Gary E. Servais, Prem Singh Virdi

Department of Ophthalmology, University of Iowa, Iowa City, Iowa, USA

Key Words. Arterial hypertension · Hard exudates · Hypertensive retinopathy · Lipid deposits · Malignant arterial hypertension · Retina

Abstract. In 60 rhesus monkeys with experimental renovascular malignant arterial hypertension (25 one-kidney and 35 two-kidney model animals), we studied the so-called 'hard exudates' or white retinal deposits in detail (by ophthalmoscopy, and stereoscopic color fundus photography and fluorescein fundus angiography, on long-term follow-up). Some manifestation of hypertensive retinopathy developed in 19 one-kidney and 19 two-kidney animals, and white deposits formed in 14 and 5 monkeys, respectively. The onset of white deposits showed no correlation to severity of arterial hypertension or of retinopathy. All eyes with white deposits had antecedent macular or retinal edema. The deposits were everchanging, taking months or even more than a year to resolve. Our study suggests that in hypertensive retinopathy the white retinal deposits are most probably the result of exudative and/or neural degenerative processes. All the available pieces of evidence indicate that it is more appropriate to call the white deposits 'lipid deposits' than 'hard exudates'.

The so-called 'hard exudates', lipid deposits or white deposits, have been well known for as long as hypertensive retinopathy has been documented, and they are said to occur frequently in malignant arterial hypertension [1]. In spite of that, it is hard to find much definite information in the literature about different aspects of these deposits in hypertensive retinopathy, particularly with respect to their association and correlation to blood pressure level or other retinal manifestations of hypertension, nor their natural history, or pathogenesis. In view of that, and since the white deposits constitute an important retinal finding in hypertensive retinopathy, we decided to investigate these lesions *clinically* in detail in our experimental studies on malignant arterial hypertension in rhesus monkeys.

Materials and Methods

Renovascular malignant arterial hypertension was produced in 60 rhesus monkeys by a modified Goldblatt's procedure. Details of our procedure to produce hypertension and methods employed for blood pressure, fundus and systemic evaluation, in this study are reported elsewhere [2]. Briefly, the animals consisted of two groups: *one-kidney, one-clip model* (25 monkeys) which had only one kidney, and that kidney was ischemic, and *two-kidney, one-clip model* (35 monkeys) that had one ischemic kidney and one normal kidney.

All monkeys were investigated by recording renal function, blood pressure (BP) and fundus changes (by direct and indirect ophthalmoscopy, color stereoscopic fundus photography, and fluorescein fundus angiography) before renal artery clamping and serially thereafter. We could reliably record only the systolic BP in the monkeys [2]. The various follow-up procedures were performed much more frequently during the initial stages and less often later, to record the evolution of the BP and fundus changes. The frequency of these procedures was determined by the severity of malignant hypertension and of fundus changes, systemic health of the animal and its ability to withstand frequent nembutal general anesthesia which is essential for doing fundus photography and fluorescein fundus angiography. These procedures were performed as often as possible to record the evolution of the fundus lesions, without detriment to the animal. Thus the follow-up for each animal was individualized.

BP and ophthalmoscopic and fluorescein fundus angiographic findings for all the monkeys were evaluated critically during the longitudinal follow-up period. The data for the various parameters were finally tabulated, collated and analyzed separately for the one-kidney and for the two-kidney model. The median (the 50th percentage point in data) and interquartile range (IQR; the difference between 75th and 25th percentage points) are given here for most of the parameters because these statistics present a better picture of the center and spread of a distribution than do the mean and standard deviation when there are extreme values in the data, as was the case in this study. The Spearman correlation coefficient and Wilcoxon rank sum test were used to determine the statistical significance.

Results

BP Hypertensive Retinopathy and Choroidopathy, and Follow-Up Period

For a proper understanding of the data on the retinal white deposits in malignant arterial hypertension in our study, and their correlation with other parameters, it is imperative to have some basic information on the arterial hypertension, follow-up period and incidence of hypertensive retinopathy and choroidopathy in these monkeys. We have discussed these at length elsewhere [2] and table 1 summarizes the data. Briefly, the normal median systolic BP in the rhesus monkeys was 120 (IQR 15) mm Hg. We decided to consider that a systolic BP of 160 mm Hg or greater was a hypertensive level. Renovascular arterial hypertension developed in all 60 monkeys. It developed significantly ($p = 0.01$) earlier in the one-kidney model than in the two-kidney model. Although there was no significant difference in the one-time highest recorded BP (either in the time it took for the BP to reach that level or in the highest level of BP recorded) in the two models, the animals of the one-kidney group developed much more rapid and more severe accelerated arterial hypertension than the two-kidney group [2]. BP findings in the two groups are summarized in table 1. Of the 25 one-kidney monkeys, 5 died within 3 weeks after surgery because of accelerated hypertension or uremia. The follow-up data for the 20 one-kidney animals that survived ≥3 weeks and for the 35 two-kidney animals is given in table 1. Some evidence of hypertensive retinopathy developed in 19 (of the 20 surviving ≥3 weeks) one-kidney and 19 two-kidney monkeys. One or another ophthalmoscopically visible lesion of hypertensive choroidopathy developed in 19 one-kidney and 14 two-kidney animals while fluorescein fundus angiographic abnormalities of the choroidal vascular bed developed in 20 and 16 monkeys respectively.

White Deposits (or So-Called 'Hard Exudates') in the Retina

In the present study, these were seen both in the macular retina and in areas of retina away from the macular region.

Table 1. Length of follow-up, BP findings and hypertensive retinopathy in one-kidney and two-kidney animals

	One-kidney group (25 monkeys)			Two-kidney group (35 monkeys)		
	range	median	IQR	range	median	IQR
Follow-up period, months	1.2–57.3[1]	9.6[1]	19.2[1]	0.7–42.3	26.4	10.5
Time interval (days) from renal artery clamping to						
Onset of hypertension	2– 43	7	3	2–115	15	18
Maximum BP recorded	2–980	110	287	8–899	124	237
Onset of hypertensive retinopathy	12– 63[2]	22[2]	17[2]	8–302[3]	64[3]	44[3]
Onset of hypertensive choroidopathy	15–133[2]	41[2]	27[2]	15–284[4]	71.5[4]	69[4]
Highest BP recorded						
BP level, in mm Hg	178–260	220	30	160–260	204	50
% Rise from baseline BP	148–245	193	46	133–237	175	26
BP (mmHg) at onset of						
Hypertensive retinopathy	164–225[2]	190[2]	21[2]	160–210[3]	178[3]	26[3]
Hypertensive choroidopathy	160–240[2]	190[2]	20[2]	160–230[4]	180[4]	30[4]

[1] In 20 animals that survived ≥3 weeks.
[2] Hypertensive retinopathy and choroidopathy both seen in 19 one-kidney monkeys.
[3] Hypertensive retinopathy seen in 19 two-kidney monkeys.
[4] Hypertensive choroidopathy seen in 14 two-kidney monkeys.

In the Macular Region

In the One-Kidney Model. White deposits in the macular region were seen in 9 (of the 19 with hypertensive retinopathy) animals, usually involving both eyes. The deposits were first seen 23–147 (median 83, IQR 12) days after the renal artery clamping when the BP was 174–240 (median 190, IQR 16) mm Hg, and retinopathy was usually of moderate severity, with ophthalmoscopically visible macular edema and retinal detachment in the macular region. On statistical analysis, there was no significant correlation between the day the white deposits first appeared and the BP or severity of retinopathy at that time. There was also no correlation between the presence or severity of these deposits and the severity or extent of retinal detachment and macular edema – some of the eyes with marked retinal detachment never developed any white deposits. Eyes without these deposits had retinopathy, macular edema and retinal detachment similar to those with the deposits, and their duration in some of the former eyes was even longer than in the latter. The retinal deposits lasted for about 3–30 (median 10, IQR 13) weeks. In a few eyes these deposits were no more than a few fine white granules while in others they were more extensive. The deposits were located in the temporal part of the macular region in 8 of the 9 animals (fig. 1a, 2) and at other sites less frequently. They generally spared the central foveolar region.

In the Two-Kidney Model. The white deposits developed in 2 of the 5 animals with macular edema in this group, 2 and 5 weeks after the onset of macular edema. The BP in these 2

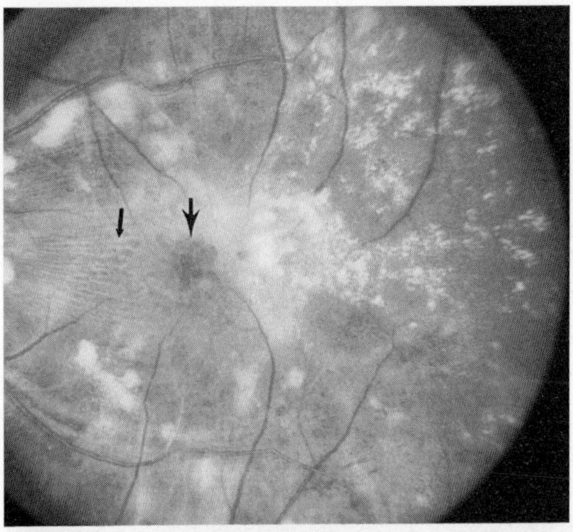

a

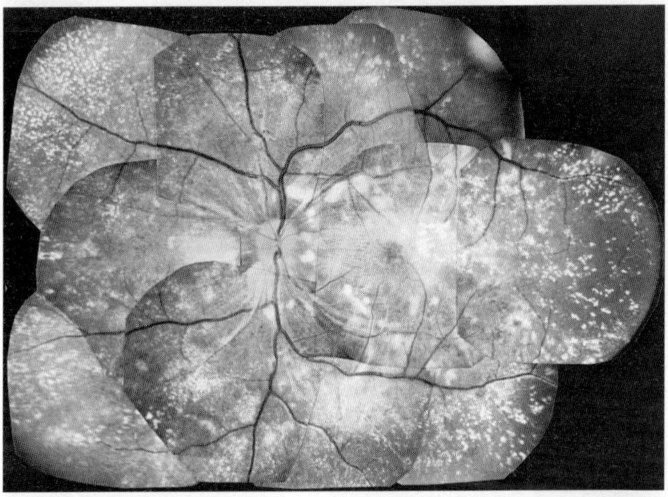

b

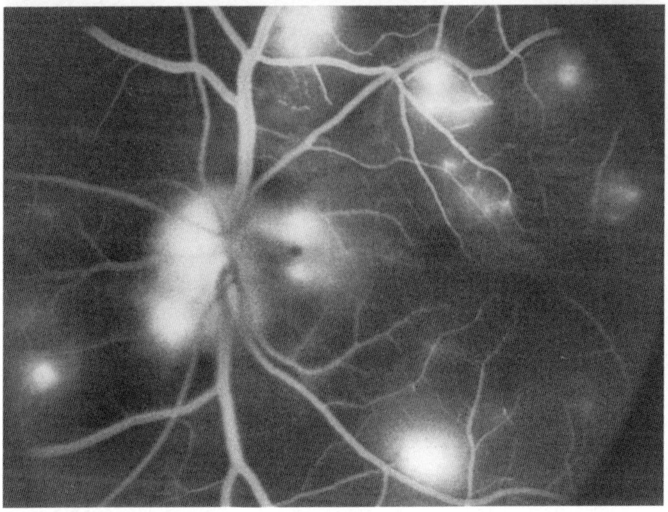

c

Fig. 1. Ophthalmoscopic (**a, b**) and fluorescein fundus angiographic (**c**) appearance of left eye in a one-kidney monkey (day 146; BP 218 mm Hg). **a** Fundus photograph of the macular region. **b** Composite fundus photograph: these show retinal arteriolar sclerosis, multiple CWSs, extensive granular white deposits in the peripheral retina, a flat serous retinal detachment in the macular region with opaque subretinal exudative deposit, marked microcystic macular edema (large arrow) and separation of retinal nerve fibers by edema (small arrow). **c** Fluorescein angiogram during the late phase showing fluorescein leaking spots due to FIPTs but no staining of the microcystic region.

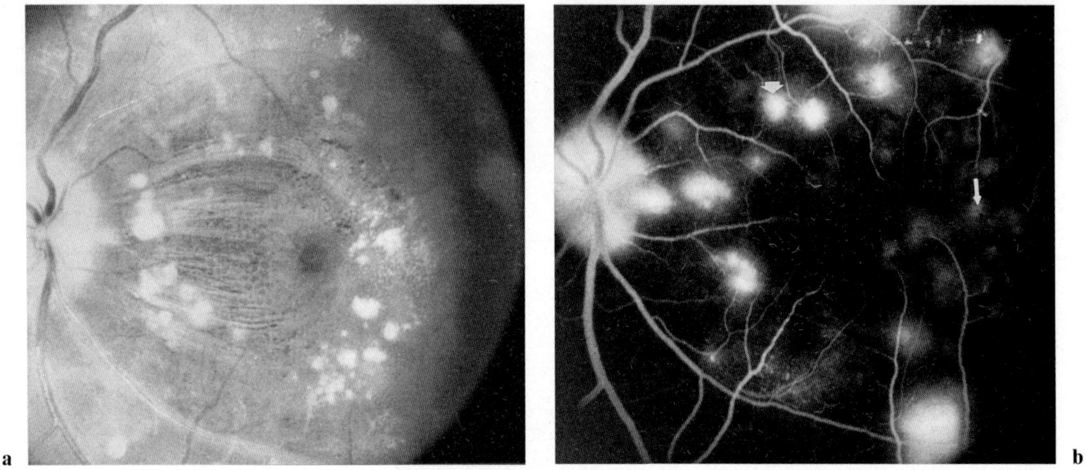

Fig. 2. Ophthalmoscopic (**a**) and fluorescein angiographic (**b**) appearance of left eye of a one-kidney monkey on day 174 with BP 212 mm Hg. Published courtesy of *Ophthalmology* 1986;93:1383–1400 [11]. **a** Fundus photograph shows marked microcystic macular edema with separation of nerve fibers by edema, foveal cyst, a few FIPTs, CWSs temporal to the optic disk, white deposits temporal to the fovea, flat serous retinal detachment of macular region associated with clear subretinal fluid, and retinal arteriolar sclerosis. **b** Fluorescein angiogram during the late phase showing multiple bright fluorescent spots corresponding to the FIPTs (large arrow) and many dull spots in temporal region of the macula due to degenerative focal choroidal lesions (small arrow), with no staining of the microcystic region and the foveal cyst.

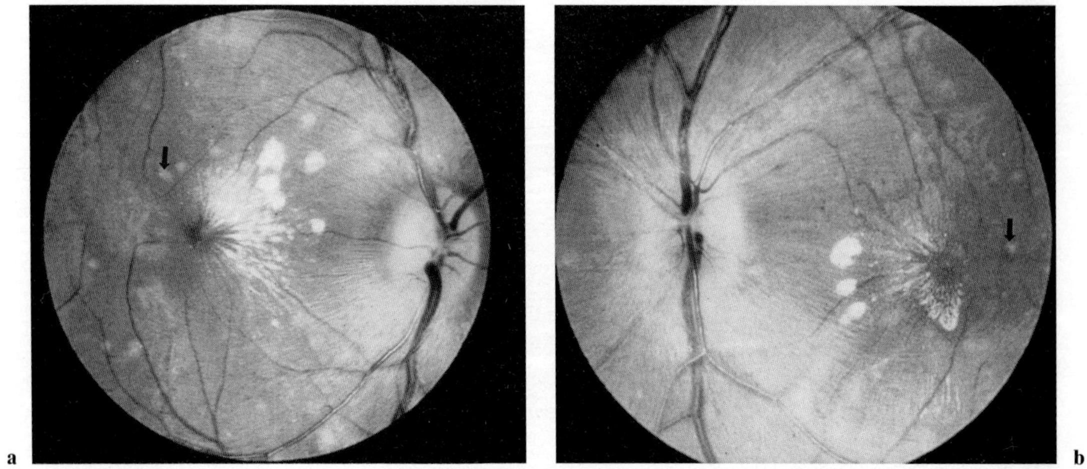

Fig. 3. Fundus photographs of both eyes of a two-kidney monkey, on day 176 with BP 190 mm Hg, show white deposits in the macular region with macular edema and a few focal retinal pigment epithelial lesions (arrow) in the temporal part of the macular region.

animals at the time of development of the deposits was 190 and 215 mm Hg, respectively. One of the two animals had marked generalized retinal edema, and neither had any retinal detachment. The macular deposits in these 2 animals were still present at the last follow-up, 1.5 and 2 years after onset.

The retinal white deposits in the macular region assumed different shapes, including that of an open Japanese fan, with its handle at the fovea (fig. 3, 4), star-shaped (fig. 5, 6) or irregular deposits (fig. 1, 2, 6).

In the Retina Outside the Macular Region

In the One-Kidney Model. These were seen in 14 of the 19 animals with hypertensive retinopathy, involving both eyes in all except 1. The white deposits first appeared 22–168 (median 69.5, IQR 34) days after the renal artery clamping, when the BP was 173–240 (median 191, IQR 24) mm Hg, and retinopathy usually of moderate severity. On statistical analysis, there was no significant correlation between the day of development of these white deposits and the BP or severity of retinopathy at that time. The deposits were constantly changing in size, shape and location, with new lesions appearing as older ones resolved. In view of the highly variable course of white deposits in different eyes and multiple factors controlling that, it is impossible to give specific data on the various constantly changing parameters of the deposits in a sample size like the present series. The white deposits varied from a few spots, as fine granular deposits, to a massive collection, usually arranged in an arc or circle (mild in 6, moderate in 4, marked in 2 and massive in 2), and the amount was similar in the two eyes of an animal. Most of the white deposits were located in the peripheral retina (fig. 1b, 7), almost always temporal to the macular region (in addition to those in the macular region, described above). Whenever there was a long-standing retinal detachment, involving the posterior pole, the white deposits were located in the attached retina just outside the boundary of the retinal detachment (fig. 7). In some eyes there were also perivascular white deposits, situated along the major retinal vessels (fig. 1b, 4a, 7).

All the eyes with white deposits had retinal detachment, mostly of the macular region with or without that of the peripapillary region. The retinal detachment almost always appeared before the white deposits; however, in the 4 animals where no white deposits developed, a similar or even total retinal detachment was seen.

All the eyes with white deposits had edema of the retina in the macular region (macular edema) for 7–56 (median 20, IQR 20) days before the development of the former. All eyes had retinopathy, including focal intraretinal periarteriolar transudates [3] and cotton-wool spots (CWSs); however, the eyes without white deposits also had similar retinal changes. Thus, apart from macular edema, there was no apparent correlation between the development of white deposits and the occurrence of various retinopathic changes.

In the Two-Kidney Model. White deposits (in the retina outside the macular region) of variable amount were seen in 5 animals, 108–1,198 (median 512, IQR 652) days after renal artery clamping when the BP was 190–220 (median 215, IQR 6) mm Hg, and there was no statistically significant correlation between the two parameters. These deposits were usually of a mild degree, located in all the animals in the peripapillary retina and in 3 of them also in the macular region. In 4 of the 5 animals these were associated with retinal edema which preceded white deposits by 1–2 months in 2 and 1 year in 1, while in the 4th animal both were

4a
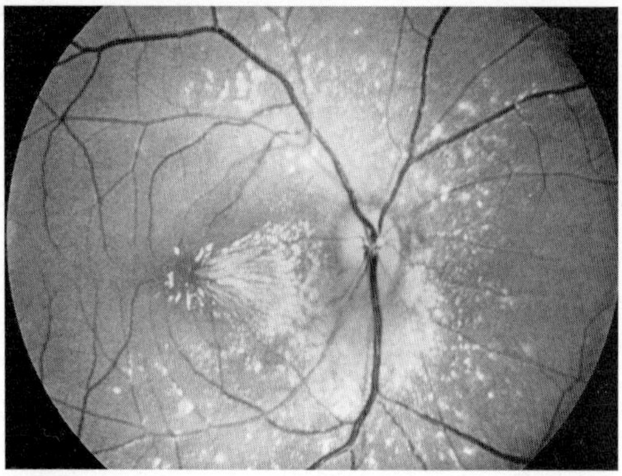
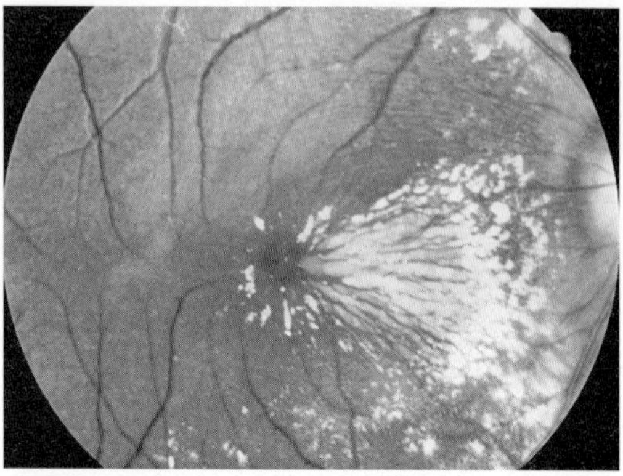
4b

5
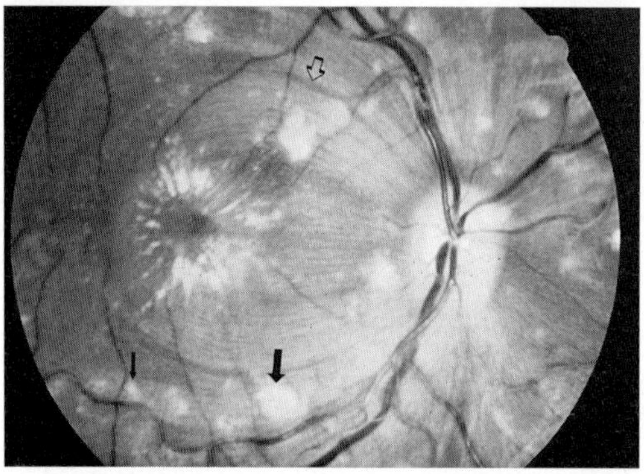
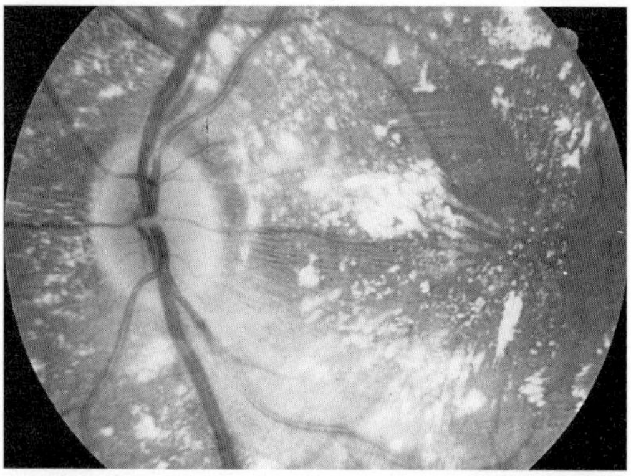
6

7a
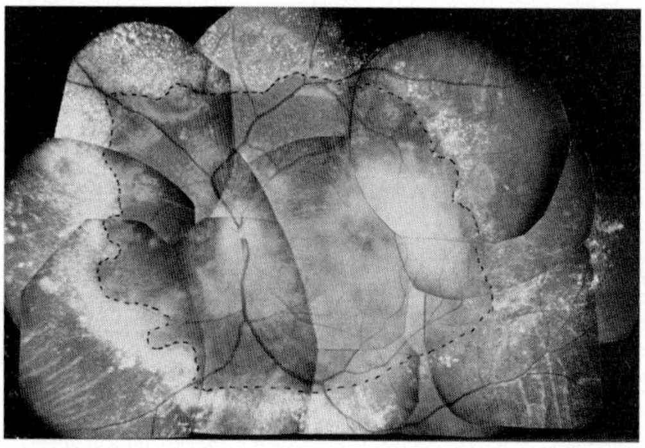
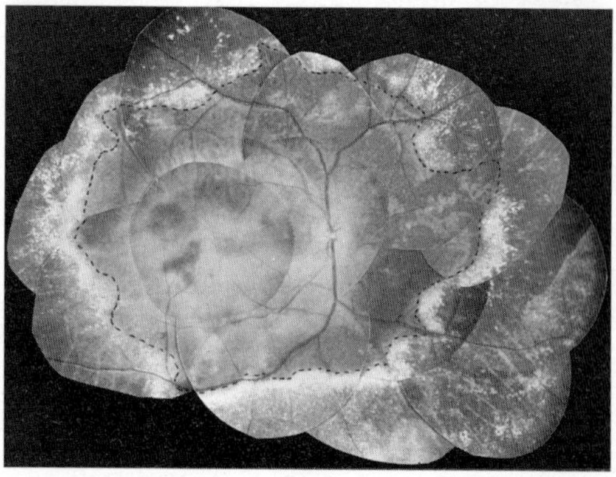
7b

Fig. 4–6. Fundus photographs of eyes of rhesus monkeys, with arterial hypertension (two-kidney model) and on atherogenic diet (not part of the series presented in this study), show extensive white deposits at the posterior pole, much more than seen in comparable hypertensive monkeys of the present series without atherogenic diet. **4b** is a magnified view of the macular region in **4a. 5** also shows serous retinal detachment in the macular region with macular edema, CWSs (large arrow), FIPTs (small arrow) and nerve fiber loss (hollow arrow).

Fig. 7. Ophthalmoscopic appearance in a one-kidney monkey. **a** Left eye on day 218 with BP 220 mm Hg. Published courtesy of *Ophthalmology* 1986;93:1383–1400 [11]. **b** Right eye on day 254 with BP 210 mm Hg. Composite fundus photographs show serous retinal detachment (outlined by a dotted line), surrounded by white deposits, and microcystic macular edema; a thick, dense layer of subretinal exudative deposit lies on the retinal pigment epithelium at the posterior pole.

observed almost simultaneously; in the remaining 1 animal a few white deposits were seen in the peripapillary retina without any associated evident retinal edema. In only 1 of these animals was foveal retinal detachment seen, about a year before the onset of white deposits. The white deposits lasted from 3 to more than 24 months.

Comments

The so-called 'hard exudates' or white retinal deposits constitute an extravascular lesion of hypertensive retinopathy, mostly consisting of deposits in the outer plexiform layer of the retina. They are said to appear commonly in malignant arterial hypertension [1], but there is little precise information in the literature on the subject of white deposits in hypertensive retinopathy. Moreover, what meager information there is on the subject of retinal white deposits in general, is mostly based on a study of these deposits in diabetic retinopathy.

Retinal White Deposits in Hypertensive Retinopathy

In the present study, about three quarters of the one-kidney eyes with hypertensive retinopathy developed white deposits in one or another part of the retina – less frequently in the macular region and posterior pole than in the more peripheral retina. When located in the macular region, the deposits were much more often in the temporal part of the foveal or macular region (fig. 1, 2) than elsewhere in the area, and usually spared the central foveolar region (fig. 1–5). We found no statistically significant correlation between the time of development of the white deposits after the renal artery clamping and the severity of arterial hypertension or of retinopathy at that time. The number and size of white deposits, both in the macular and extramacular regions, varied from a few fine white granules to a massive aggregate. The deposits were ever-changing, and took many months or even more than a year to clear, most probably because of their location in the avascular outer plexiform layer of the retina. Classically, white deposits in the macula in malignant hypertension are described as a 'macular star'. The deposition of material within the radially oriented fibers of Henle's layer in the macula is said to account for the radial arrangement of these deposits like 'rays of light emanating from a star' (fig. 3–5). However, in the present study of experimentally induced malignant hypertension, white macular deposits assumed a variety of shapes including an open Japanese fan, with its 'handle' at the fovea (fig. 3, 4), a complete star (fig. 5, 6), or irregularly scattered deposits without a radial orientation (fig. 1, 2, 6). Thus the term 'macular star' for these is not always valid. Although most macular white deposits are seen in eyes with macular edema in malignant hypertension, the reason for the location and development of the deposits is still not understood.

In our study, we did not see white macular deposits without antecedent macular edema; however, macular edema did not always result in white deposits. The white deposits may appear while retinal hemorrhages and CWSs are clearing.

Pathogenesis of Retinal White Deposits in Hypertensive Retinopathy

This is still ill-understood, as is also the case with white deposits in other retinopathies. The pathogenesis of white deposits in general has been explained by the following three theories: exudation, retinal cell injury, and resolution of retinal hemorrhages.

Exudative phenomenon: the most widely accepted view is that they are derived from the circulating blood, and caused by undue retinal vascular permeability, so that they can be considered a manifestation of retinal microangiopathy and breakdown of the blood-retinal barrier, i.e. exudative retinopathy. It is thought that ultimately the fluid part of the exudate is reabsorbed, leaving inspissated remains which are partly taken up by the phagocytes (microglial cells). Most of the views are based on studies of white deposits seen in diabetic retinopathy. Yanoff [4], on histopathology in diabetic retinopathy, found that macrophages (histiocytes) with foamy or clear cytoplasm are seen within and surrounding the deposits, most likely engulfing and removing the material; according to him, their location in the outer plexiform layer is most probably due to edema fluid pooling in an avascular area where it cannot be reabsorbed into the capillary bed; he further added that glial-neuronal cell breakdown products (see below) are likely additional constituents of these deposits. Ashton [5] postulated that in malignant hypertension the high lipid content of the retinal exudates is largely hematogenous in origin and to a small degree a by-product of hypoxic retinal tissue (see below). He further added that these exudates, partly engulfed by macrophages, collect in the outer retina where they may form the macular star; according to him, a shallow retinal detachment is not uncommon.

Retinal cell injury: Yanoff [4] and Ashton [5], as mentioned above, were of the opinion that glial-neuronal degeneration contributed only to a small extent to the white deposits. In contrast to that, some researchers believe that the by-products of degenerated retinal cells contribute to what is clinically seen as white deposits. Houston and Wise [6], in circinate retinopathy, postulated that the white retinal deposits represent fats liberated from fatty degeneration of the dead retinal cells and that phagocytic cells (microglial cells) ingest the fat, migrate to the border of the lesion and aggregate there, forming the deposits which are eventually absorbed [6]. Bloodworth [7], in diabetic retinopathy, denied a causal relationship between white deposits and vascular disease, and suggested that the deposits were due to neuronal and glial cell degeneration 'perhaps associated with some plasma proteins'. Gass [8] stated that the absence of fluorescein leakage from the macular capillaries in the presence of white deposits in the macular region, and the failure of these deposits to stain with fluorescein, suggest that they may be, in part at least, products of retinal tissue breakdown rather than serous exudate derived from retinal vessels. However, he stated that one cannot exclude the possibility that they are inspissated exudative products which stem from extramacular retinal vessels and have gravitated centrally into the outer plexiform layer which is most prominent in the macular region.

Due to phagocytosis of the retinal hemorrhages in hypertensive retinopathy: Leishman [9] put forward this view. However, the deposits are not related topographically to either hemorrhages or CWSs. This hypothesis seems the least likely explanation. Our study did not provide any evidence in support of this view.

The clinical findings of our experimental studies on fundus changes in malignant hypertension have provided some important clues to the pathogenesis of the white deposits in malignant hypertension. Our various observations suggest the following two mechanisms for the development of white deposits in hypertensive retinopathy:

White Deposits Exudative in Nature

This is suggested by several pieces of evidence from the present study and these include the following:

(1) All eyes with white deposits had retinal detachment (mostly of the macular region) and macular edema. From this, it would seem logical to postulate that macular edema and retinal detachment have something to do with the formation of these deposits or are connected in some way.

What, then, is the cause of macular edema and retinal detachment in these eyes with malignant arterial hypertension – is the macular edema and retinal detachment of retinal vascular origin or of some other? In the past, retinal edema and associated serous retinal detachment were usually ascribed to increased retinal vascular permeability and leakage of the serum contents into the retinal tissue. During the acute phase of hypertensive retinopathy, with focal intraretinal periarteriolar transudates (FIPTs) [3] and marked generalized retinal edema, there is irrefutable clinical, fluorescein fundus angiographic and histopathologic evidence of serum leakage from the retinal vessels; and our study also revealed that [3]. Later on, in the course of hypertensive retinopathy, however, our studies on fluorescein fundus angiography revealed no noticeable retinal vascular leakage or microangiopathy or staining of the white deposits in these eyes when macular edema and white deposits were present; this was also reported by Gass [8] in his fluorescein fundus angiographic studies on patients with hypertensive retinopathy and white deposits. This makes it most unlikely that exudation from the retinal vascular bed is the main cause of macular edema and white deposits. It could be argued that fluorescein fundus angiography may not be a sensitive enough test to reveal the subtle leakage from the retinal vascular bed; this was shown by Tso and Shih [10] in their studies on experimental postcataract extraction macular edema in monkeys where, in spite of obvious disruption of blood-retinal barrier on light and electron microscopy by a horseradish peroxidase tracer technique, no such disruption was seen by fluorescein fundus angiography. The possibility of such minute leakage cannot be ruled out, but it could not produce the degree of macular edema and retinal detachment seen in the eyes of the present study when the white deposits were seen. Therefore one has to look elsewhere for the cause of serous retinal detachment and associated macular edema.

Our studies on hypertensive choroidopathy [11] (supported by clinical observations in patients with malignant hypertension and preeclampsia) strongly indicate that the retinal detachment in these eyes is essentially due to leakage of fluid from the choriocapillaris into the subretinal space; this is produced by breakdown of the blood-retinal barrier in the retinal pigment epithelium by hypoxia or ischemia of the latter, secondary to choroidal ischemia seen in hypertensive choroidopathy [11]. Our histopathological studies using horseradish peroxidase in hypertensive choroidopathy further revealed that the subretinal fluid is derived from the choriocapillaris and the detached retina imbibes subretinal fluid [11]; the latter happens because there is no physical or physiologic barrier to prevent detached retina from acting like a sponge, so that most probably the retinal edema in these eyes is at least partly, if not entirely, due to the associated serous retinal detachment [11]. This is further indicated by the fact that, in about two thirds of these animals, ophthalmoscopically visible macular edema (as revealed by examination of stereoscopic fundus photographs) developed at the same time as the serous detachment; in about one third retinal detachment developed before the ophthalmoscopically evident macular edema, and macular edema occasionally preceded ophthalmoscopically demonstrable macular retinal detachment. When macular edema preceded retinal detachment, the possibility is that the fluid leakage from the choroid, via the hypoxic retinal pigment epithelium, was too slight to produce clinically visible retinal detachment, but enough to produce edema in the overlying macular retina. Ashton [5] also found not uncommonly a shallow retinal detachment in eyes with hypertensive retinopathy and retinal exudates. In our study, most of the eyes with macular edema showed, on ophthalmoscopy, cyst-like accumulations of intraretinal fluid, almost invariably without retinal microangiopathy or leakage from the retinal vascular bed on fluorescein fundus angiography (fig. 1c, 2b); this would further support the concept that the fluid may be coming from the choroid rather than from the retinal vessels.

These findings strongly indicate that usually neither the macular edema nor the white deposits are primarily due to exudation from the retinal circulation; however, the possibility of a minor contribution by exudation from the retinal vessels cannot be ruled out. In these eyes, leakage from the choroidal circulation appears to be the major source of the exudation in the subretinal space as well as in the retinal tissue (secondary to seepage of subretinal fluid into the retinal tissue). Likewise, many of the white deposits seen in these eyes may have been derived from the subretinal fluid that gained entrance from the choroidal vessels rather than the retinal vessels. Once the exudative fluid, derived from the subretinal fluid, enters the retina, it is impossible to distinguish it from that which may be derived from the retinal vessels. Similarly, the white deposits derived from this exudative fluid in the retina would assume ophthalmoscopic and morphological features as if these were of retinal origin. Free lipids have been found in the choroidal stroma [12] and this is evidence of increased permeability of the choroidal vascular bed in malignant hypertension.

(2) In our ongoing studies in rhesus monkeys with combined experimental arterial hypertension and experimentally induced hyperlipidemia and atherosclerosis (produced by an atherogenic diet), we have found a much higher incidence and more extensive distribution of these deposits (fig. 4–6) than in hypertensive animals with normal serum lipids. Similarly, in our prospective clinical studies on patients with retinal vein occlusion, we have observed that diabetics tend to have a much higher incidence of white deposits than nondiabetics. These findings indicate that when the blood-retinal barrier breaks down (whether in the retinal vessels or in the retinal pigment epithelium), serum with high lipids leaks into the retinal tissue, resulting in exaggerated white deposits.

The above findings indicate that exudation plays an important role in the pathogenesis of the retinal white deposits in malignant hypertension, and that the deposits are derived from the serum exudation. There is strong evidence that the choroidal vascular bed is the major source of the exudation (and likewise of the retinal white deposits), with possibly a small contribution from the retinal vascular bed.

Gass [13] suggested that macular star in most cases is related to exudation occurring in the optic nerve head, and postulated that exudate from vessels in the depths of the optic nerve head leaks into peripapillary subretinal space and along the outer plexiform layer into the macular area. Our studies showed no evidence that white deposits in the macular region in malignant arterial hypertension are related in any way to exudation occurring in the optic nerve head.

There is ample evidence in the literature that retinal and subretinal exudates contain lipids as well as other materials such as glycoproteins, because classical histopathologic studies on these exudates demonstrate their affinity for the periodic acid-Schiff (PAS) stain. Our preliminary histopathologic studies in these eyes confirmed this. This is to be expected, because breakdown of the blood-retinal barrier permits the escape of all plasma constituents into the exudate.

White Deposits a By-Product of Degenerated Retinal Cells

Exudation does not explain all the features of retinal white deposits seen in this study. For example, in the present series, in eyes with long-standing retinal detachment, we often found marked amounts of white deposits located in the attached retina just outside the boundary of the retinal detachment (as seen in fig. 7), without any evidence of associated retinal microangiopathy or, on fluorescein angiography, leakage in the detached or attached retina or staining of the white deposits. This would suggest some other mechanism, in addition to or unrelated to exudation, causing the development of retinal white deposits. Retinal cell injury has been postulated as the source of the white deposits by a number of researchers in the past [4–8]. This is a reasonable view, because, for example, plasmalemma of retinal cells is rich in lipids, and damage to the outer segments of photoreceptors (seen in long-standing retinal detachment in the present study) or irreversible retinal cell injury (from chronic hypoxia, chronic ischemia or chronic edema) would permit phagocytic cells to collect the released lipids and deposit them at the edge of the injury zone. In the present study, it was not uncommon to see the deposits disappear before the resolution of the retinal detachment; the reason for this may possibly be that once the degeneration of the outer retinal tissue and/or other retinal cells is complete, there is no further retinal degeneration and hence no more release of lipids, so that the retinal detachment may persist without white deposits. This would suggest that degeneration of the outer retinal tissue associated with retinal detachment and/or retinal cell degeneration from hypoxia or chronic edema may be partly, if not entirely, responsible for the white deposits in these eyes. The other possibility is that retinal ischemia (due to retinal and/or choroidal ischemia) in hypertensive retinopathy could account for the clinically swollen retina (without true edema and accumulation of extracellular fluid); in that case, a by-product of hypoxic retinal tissue could produce white deposits, as suggested by Ashton [5].

There are, however, some problems with the hypothesis that retinal white deposits are by-products of retinal cell injury and degeneration. For example, patients' eyes with long-standing retinal detachment do not usually develop white deposits; also a few eyes with retinal detachment in our study did not develop white deposits. The other problem with this hypotheses is that we do not yet have definite proof that retinal white deposits are a by-product of the degenerated retinal cells.

On balance, one has to consider this a plausible but unproven explanation for the mechanism of white deposits, because there is some evidence of its occurring in our study, there are logical reasons to believe that it does occur, and it has been postulated by most authors [4–8] who have discussed the subject in the past, since exudation does not explain the pathogenesis of white deposits in every case.

It is a common clinical observation that the white deposits in various types of retinopathy are almost always located in the healthy retina adjacent to the edematous or unhealthy retina. In the eyes of the present study, the retina in the macular region, because of chronic edema and detachment, was unhealthy, which may be an important reason why most of the white deposits were located in the peripheral retina, usually temporal to the macular region, with the macular region usually not showing extensive deposits. Similarly, another possible reason for the location of retinal white deposits at the margin of retinal detachment may be that in the normal retina around the detachment the fluid contents of the exudates may be removed by the normal retinal and choroidal vessels – a mechanism similar to that seen in circinate retinopathy and subretinal choroidal neovascularization.

Conclusion

The available pieces of evidence in the literature as well as in the present study indicate that *in hypertensive retinopathy* the white deposits are most probably the result of exudative as well as neural degenerative processes, individually or collectively. Which is the predominant factor we do not yet know; it may well vary from eye to eye and/or from time to time. We cannot comment to what extent findings from white deposits in hypertensive retinopathy can be extrapolated to white deposits in other types of retinopathy and vice versa, because the basic pathologic lesions in various types of retinopathy are not identical.

Terminology

The terminology of this lesion is very confusing. Since all the available evidence indicates that the major constituent of these deposits is always lipid, and that these white deposits may develop in the absence of exudation, it would be more suitable to call them 'lipid deposits' than 'hard exudates', as the latter term in some cases may be a misnomer.

Acknowledgments

We are grateful to Dr. Robert F. Woolson and Dr. Marie R. Klugman of the Department of Preventive Medicine (Biostatistics) for their help with statistical analyses of the data, to Dr. Robert Folberg, Ocular Pathologists in the Department of Ophthalmology for valuable suggestions, to Mrs. Ellen Ballas and Mrs. Georgiane Parkes-Perret for their secretarial help, to Mr. James Swaner for the technical help, and to the Photography Department for the illustrations. This research was supported by a research grant from the National Eye Institute (EY-1576) and in part by an unrestricted grant from Research to Prevent Blindness, Inc., and from Alcon Research Institute.

References

1 Duke-Elder S, Dobree JH: System of Ophthalmology – Diseases of the retina, vol. 10. London, Kimpton, 1967, pp 331–332, 340.
2 Hayreh SS, Servais GE, Virdi PS, et al: Fundus lesions in malignant hypertension. III. Arterial blood pressure, biochemical and fundus changes. Ophthalmology 1986;93:45–59.
3 Hayreh SS, Servais GE, Virdi PS: Fundus lesions in malignant hypertension. IV. Focal intraretinal periarteriolar transudates. Ophthalmology 1986; 93:60–73.
4 Yanoff M: Ocular pathology of diabetes mellitus. Am J Ophthalmol 1969;67:21–38.
5 Ashton N: The eye in malignant hypertension. Trans Am Acad Ophthalmol Otolaryngol 1972;76:17–40.
6 Houston WR, Wise GN: Circinate retinopathy. Arch Ophthalmol 1957;58:777–782.
7 Bloodworth JMB: Diabetic retinopathy. Diabetes 1962;11:1–22.
8 Gass JDM: A fluorescein angiographic study of macular dynsfunction secondary to retinal vascular

disease. III. Hypertensive retinopathy. Arch Ophthalmol 1968;80:569–582.
9 Leishman R: The eye in general vascular disease – Hypertension and arteriosclerosis. Br J Ophthalmol 1957;41:461–701.
10 Tso MOM, Shih C-Y: Experimental macular edema after lens extraction. Invest Ophthalmol Vis Sci 1977;16:381–392.
11 Hayreh SS, Servais GE, Virdi PS: Fundus lesions in malignant hypertension. VI. Hypertensive choroidopathy. Ophthalmology 1986;93:1383–1400.
12 Gasteiger H: Über histologische Befunde am Auge bei Nieren- and Blutdruckveränderungen. Klin Monatsbl Augenheilkd 1937;99:604–625.
13 Gass JDM: Diseases of the optic nerve that may simulate macular disease. Trans Am Acad Ophthalmol Otolaryngol 1977;83:OP-763–770.

Dr. S. S. Hayreh
Department of Ophthalmology
University of Iowa Hospitals and Clinics
Iowa City, IA 52242 (USA)

Ophthalmologica 1989;198:230–246

Macular Lesions in Malignant Arterial Hypertension

Sohan Singh Hayreh, Gary E. Servais, Prem Singh Virdi
Department of Ophthalmology, University of Iowa, Iowa City, Iowa, USA

Key Words. Arterial hypertension · Cystoid macular edema · Edema · Lipid deposits · Macula · Malignant arterial hypertension · Retina · Retinal pigment epithelial

Abstract. We produced experimental renovascular malignant arterial hypertension by a modified Goldblatt's procedure in 60 rhesus monkeys (25 one-kidney model and 35 two-kidney model), and studied various macular lesions by detailed serial ophthalmoscopy, and stereoscopic color fundus photography and fluorescein fundus angiography on a long-term follow-up. The various lesions which developed in the macular region included retinal edema, cystic retinal changes, serous retinal detachment, retinal pigment epithelial changes (initially acute focal and later degenerative lesions), and lipid deposits. In addition to these, the usual retinal lesions associated with hypertensive retinopathy, e.g., focal intraretinal periarteriolar transudates, cotton-wool spots and retinal hemorrhages, were also frequently seen in the macular retina. Findings on the various lesions are described in detail, and the pathogenesis of macular edema in malignant arterial hypertension is discussed.

Classical textbook descriptions of hypertensive retinopathy, apart from the presence of 'macular star', make virtually no mention of any macular involvement in patients with malignant arterial hypertension. In sharp contrast to that, our recent detailed, systematic experimental studies on renovascular malignant arterial hypertension showed frequent involvement of the macular region. This discrepancy prompted us to study macular lesions in malignant arterial hypertension in detail.

Materials and Methods

We produced renovascular arterial hypertension in 60 rhesus monkeys. This was done by a modified Goldblatt's procedure where the left renal artery was clamped, by the method described in detail elsewhere [1]. Very briefly, there were two models of hypertension: 25 monkeys of the *one-kidney, one-clip model* had the left renal artery clamped and nephrectomy on the right side, and 35 animals belonging to the *two-kidney, one-clip model* had the left renal artery clamped and the right kidney normal. All the animals were examined serially to record renal function, blood pressure (BP) and fundus changes (by direct and indirect ophthalmoscopy, color stereoscopic fundus photography, and fluorescein fundus angiography) before renal artery clamping and sequentially thereafter. Detailed information about the materials and methods employed in this study are reported in a previous publication [1]. We could record only the systolic BP by the auscultatory method used [1]. The various follow-up procedures to record the evolution of the BP and fundus changes were individualized for each monkey, usually performed much more frequently during the initial stages and, less often later, depending upon the severity of arterial hypertension and fundus lesions, the general health of the monkey and its ability to withstand the stress of the nembutal general anesthesia required for fundus photography and fluorescein fundus angiography. We critically studied BP and ophthalmoscopic and fluorescein fundus angiographic findings for all the monkeys during the longitudinal follow-up period.

The data obtained from our study on the BP and various types of fundus change during the follow-up were finally collated and analyzed separately for the one-kidney and the two-kidney model, using several statistical procedures. For the various parameters, we calculated the median (the 50th percentage point in data) and interquartile range (IQR; the difference between the 75th and 25th percentage points) because when there are extreme values in the data, as was the case in this study, median and IQR give a better picture of the center and spread of a distribution than do the mean and standard deviation. We determined statistical significance by using the Spearman correlation coefficient and Wilcoxon rank sum test.

Results

BP, Hypertensive Retinopathy and Choroidopathy, and Follow-Up Period

To correlate macular changes in malignant arterial hypertension with the BP level, duration of hypertension and incidence of hypertensive retinopathy and choroidopathy, it is essential to have some basic information about these parameters; we have discussed these at length elsewhere [1] and table 1 summarizes the data. Briefly, in rhesus monkeys the normal median systolic BP is 120 (IQR 15) mm Hg and all animals with BP of ≥160 mm Hg were considered hypertensive. All the 60 monkeys in this study developed renovascular malignant arterial hypertension, with one-kidney animals developing it significantly ($p = 0.01$) earlier than the two-kidney ones. One-kidney monkeys developed much more rapid and more severe hypertension than the two-kidney animals; however, there was no significant difference between the two models of hypertension in the one-time highest recorded BP (either in the time it took for the BP to reach the highest level or in the level of BP recorded). Five of the 25 one-kidney monkeys died within 3 weeks after renal artery clamping from complications of accelerated hypertension or uremia. Some evidence of hypertensive retinopathy developed in 19 one-kidney monkeys (out of the 20 surviving ≥3 weeks) and 19 of the 35 two-kidney monkeys. One or another ophthalmoscopically visible lesion of hypertensive choroidopathy developed in 19 one-kidney and 14 two-kidney animals while fluorescein fundus angiographic abnormalities of the choroidal vascular bed developed in 20 and 16 monkeys respectively.

Macular Retinal Edema

In the one-kidney model, macular edema was seen in 16 animals. In the remaining 3 (1 of them followed for about 2 months and the remaining 2 for more than 3 years) no ophthalmoscopically or angiographically demonstrable macular edema was ever seen, in spite of other evidence of retinopathy. Macular edema was first seen 16–168 (median 36, IQR 54) days after renal artery clamping, when the BP was 160–238 (median 190, IQR 24.5) mm Hg. In the 3 animals without macular edema, the BPs were 198, 205 and 230 mm Hg. The time of onset of macular edema showed no statistically significant correlation with either the level of

Table 1. Length of follow-up, BP findings and hypertensive retinopathy in one-kidney and two-kidney animals

	One-kidney group (25 monkeys)			Two-kidney group (35 monkeys)		
	range	median	IQR	range	median	IQR
Follow-up period, months	1.2–57.3[1]	9.6[1]	19.2[1]	0.7–42.3	26.4	10.5
Time interval (days) from renal artery clamping to						
Onset of hypertension	2– 43	7	3	2–115	15	18
Maximum BP recorded	2–980	110	287	8–899	124	237
Onset of hypertensive retinopathy	12– 63[2]	22[2]	17[2]	8–302[3]	64[3]	44[3]
Onset of hypertensive choroidopathy	15–133[2]	41[2]	27[2]	15–284[4]	71.5[4]	69[4]
Highest BP recorded						
BP level, in mm Hg	178–260	220	30	160–260	204	50
% Rise from baseline BP	148–245	193	46	133–237	175	26
BP (mmHg) at onset of						
Hypertensive retinopathy	164–225[2]	190[2]	21[2]	160–210[3]	178[3]	26[3]
Hypertensive choroidopathy	160–240[2]	190[2]	20[2]	160–230[4]	180[4]	30[4]

1 In 20 animals that survived >3 weeks.
2 Hypertensive retinopathy and choroidopathy both seen in 19 one-kidney monkeys.
3 Hypertensive retinopathy seen in 19 two-kidney monkeys.
4 Hypertensive choroidopathy seen in 14 two-kidney monkeys.

hypertension or the severity of retinopathy at that time. When macular edema was at its maximum in these animals, in 7 animals it was of marked severity, while in the remaining 9 it was mild, moderate or difficult to assess (equal numbers of animals in the three groups). At this stage, the BP was 175–240 (median 198, IQR 14.5) mm Hg. In 9 animals, the severity of macular edema corresponded with the severity of retinopathy, but not in the rest. When the macular edema was most marked, its severity had a significant correlation with the severity of cotton-wool spots (CWSs) ($p = 0.05$) and focal intraretinal periarteriolar transudates (FIPTs) [2] ($p = 0.01$).

In the two-kidney model, retinal and macular edema was seen in only 5 animals, in 34–133 (median 73, IQR 55) days, with a BP of 178–214 (median 188, IQR 32) mm Hg. The retinal edema involved the peripapillary retina and macular region in 4 and was much more extensive and marked in one.

One of the early ophthalmoscopic signs of macular edema was a change of the fovea to a yellowish color, usually surrounded by an opaque ring – these changes were in the deepest layers of the retina (fig. 1). Fluorescein fundus angiography revealed no appreciable leakage of the dye into the macular retina to correspond with macular edema. The macular

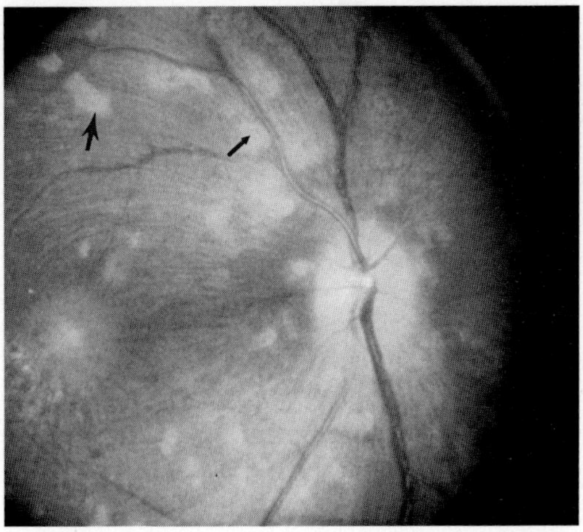

Fig. 1. Fundus photograph of right eye of a monkey with BP 190 mm Hg 90 days after renal artery clamping, showing macular edema, mild serous macular retinal detachment with subfoveal proteinaceous fluid, CWSs (large arrow) and FIPTs (along the retinal arterioles; small arrow).

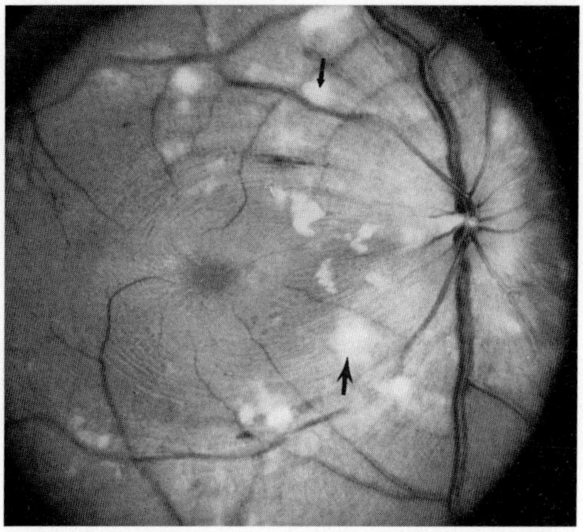

Fig. 2. Fundus photograph of right eye of a monkey with BP 190 mm Hg on day 83, showing moderate serous macular retinal detachment with proteinaceous subretinal fluid, marked macular retinal edema with mild microcystic change and separation of nerve fibers by edema, CWSs (large arrow), FIPTs (along the retinal arterioles; small arrow), and a few fine granular lipid deposits in temporal part of the foveal retina.

edema at first increased in severity, then remained stable for a variable length of time and thereafter started to resolve gradually. In about two thirds of the animals of the one-kidney group, the macular edema resolved during follow-up, having lasted for about 2–8 (median 4.25) months.

Cystoid Macular Edema

In the one-kidney model, almost all eyes with macular edema which were followed up for an adequate length of time developed variable degrees of cystoid change in the macular retina (fig. 2–7). It was first detected 22–229 (median 80.5, IQR 54) days after the renal artery clamping, with a BP of 164–245 (median 194.5, IQR 16) mm Hg. The onset of cystoid macular edema (CME) showed no statistically significant correlation with the level of hypertension or severity of retinopathy. *In the two-kidney model,* CME developed in 3 of the 5 animals with retinal edema.

The initial cystoid change was in the foveal region, varying from a fine microcystic change (fig. 2–4) to a foveal cyst (fig. 5–7). The retinopathy was usually of moderate degree at this stage. In the one-kidney model, development of CME showed no positive correlation with the severity of macular edema preceding the CME. There was also no definite relationship between the severity of CME and of associated serous retinal detachment. Fluorescein fundus angiography never revealed appreciable late staining of the microcysts in this study (fig. 3, 4, 7) although a few of the foveal cysts showed a faint late staining (fig. 5, 6).

Foveal cyst developed in almost all the eyes followed for a sufficient length of time

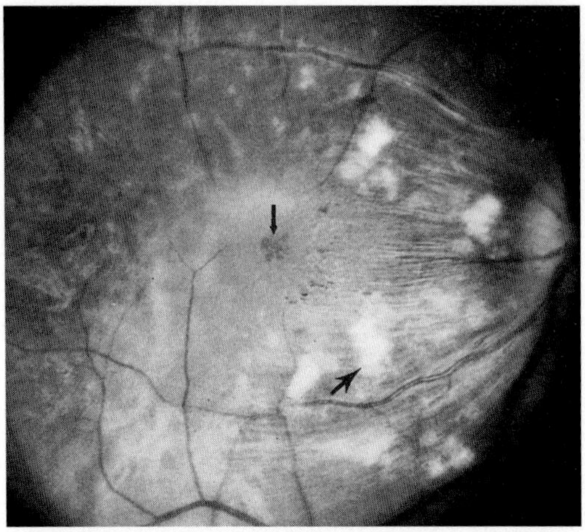

a

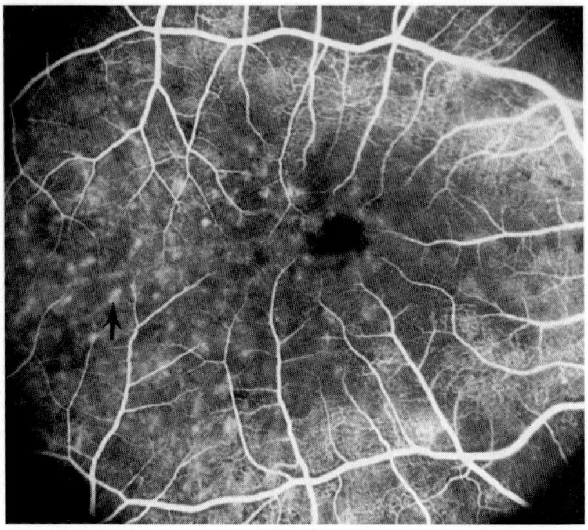

b

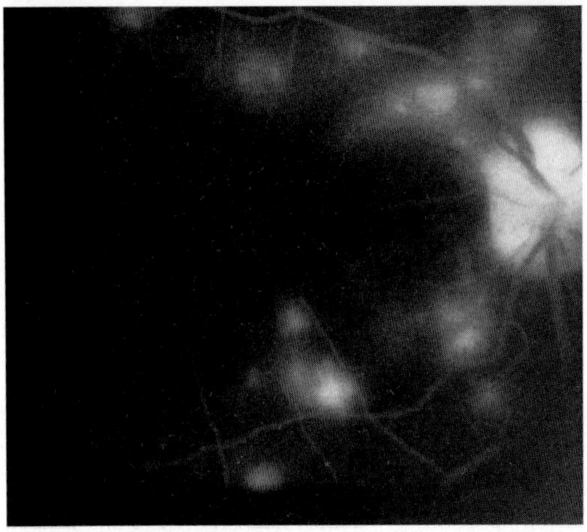

c

Fig. 3. Right eye of a monkey with BP 180 mm Hg on day 111. **a** Fundus photograph showing mild serous macular retinal detachment with proteinaceous subretinal fluid in the center, macular edema with microcystic change in the foveal region (small arrow) and separation of nerve fibers by edema, and CWSs (large arrow). Published courtesy of *Ophthalmology* 1986;93:1383–1400 [3a]. **b, c** Fluorescein angiograms during retinal arteriovenous (**b**) and late (**c**) phases, showing absence of fluorescence in the microcystic region in both phases, punctate fluorescent spots temporal to the fovea (arrow) in **b** due to focal degenerative retinal pigment epithelial (RPE) lesions, and the fluorescent spots in **c** due to leakage from the FIPTs.

(fig. 5–7); in a few eyes the cyst disappeared later on, but in the majority it persisted till the end of follow-up. In addition, there was microcystic change, usually located in the perifoveal retina; less often, it was more extensive. Separation of the nerve fibers by edema [usually in the retina between the fovea and disk (fig. 2–7), and once in a while elsewhere] was seen in about one third of the eyes of the one-kidney model. Rarely, an eye developed a foveal hole.

Macular Serous Retinal Detachment

The findings on this topic are described at length elsewhere [3a], and are briefly summarized here.

In the one-kidney model, 16 of the 19 animals developed macular serous retinal detachment (fig. 2–8), involving either the entire macular region (in 12 monkeys), or only the foveal area (in 3), or situated between the fovea and optic disk only (in 1). At onset the macular serous retinal detachment was invar-

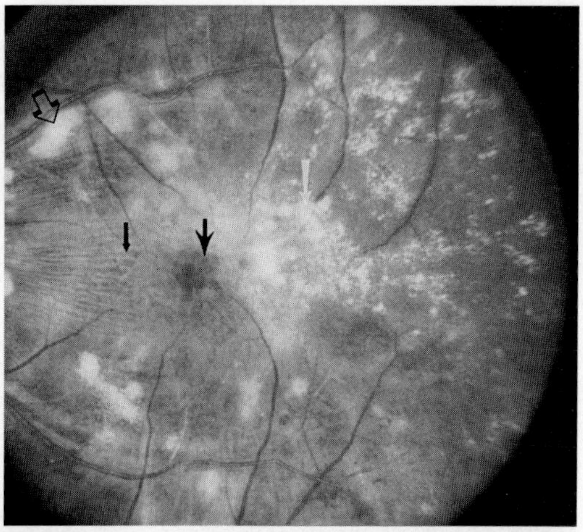
a

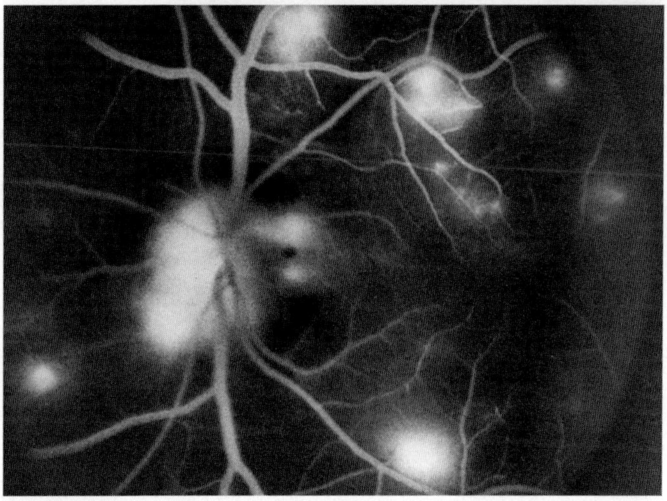
b

Fig. 4. Left eye of a monkey with BP 218 mm Hg on day 146. **a** Fundus photograph showing mild serous macular retinal detachment with subretinal proteinaceous deposits, macular edema with microcystic change in the foveal region (large arrow) and separation of nerve fibers by edema (small arrow), lipid deposits (white arrow), and CWSs (hollow arrow). **b** Fluorescein angiogram during the late phase showing leakage of dye from the FIPTs but none in the CWSs and the microcystic region.

iably bilateral and usually similar in the two eyes. The detachment varied from flat and mild (in about two thirds) to moderate (in the rest). The detachment first appeared within 53 (median) days after the renal artery clamping when the median BP was 193 mm Hg. When the detachment developed, 3 of the monkeys had no retinopathy (except for the presence of FIPTs in 2 of the 3; fig. 8), with no definite relationship apparent between the two, indicating that the serous retinal detachment was not secondary to the retinopathy. In contrast to that, all eyes with serous retinal detachment of the macular region had evidence of ischemia of the underlying choroid because all of them had already had choroidal circulatory disturbances for a variable length of time (fig. 9); 13 monkeys showed frank ischemic retinal pigment epithelial (RPE) lesions (fig. 5, 6), and in the rest either the retinal pigment epithelium (RPE) was masked by an exudative serous retinal detachment or there were no ophthalmo-

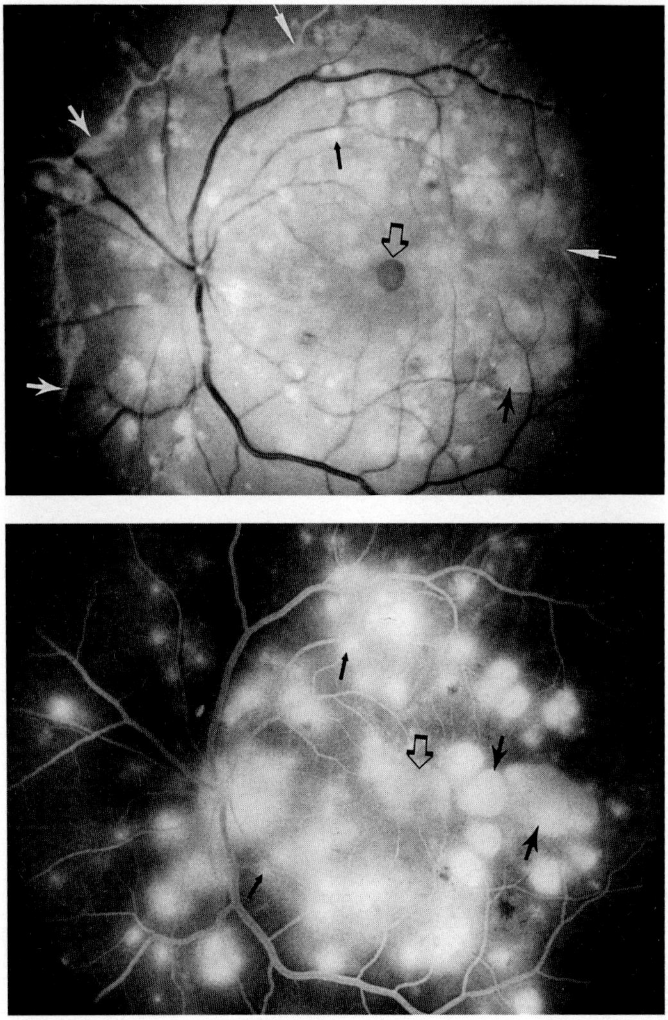

a

b

Fig. 5. Left eye of a monkey with BP 198 mm Hg on day 50. **a** Fundus photograph showing serous retinal detachment of posterior pole with clear subretinal fluid (note the demarcation line outlining the detachment; white arrow), multiple acute focal RPE lesions (large arrow), foveal cyst (hollow arrow), and multiple FIPTs (along the retinal arterioles; small arrow). Published courtesy of *Ophthalmology* 1986;93: 1383–1400 [3a]. **b** Fluorescein angiogram during the late phase showing fluorescein leakage in the FIPTs (small arrows) and acute focal RPE lesions (large arrows), with staining of the foveal cyst (hollow arrow).

scopically visible lesions (presumably the ischemic RPE lesions were too subtle to be seen opthalmoscopically).

The macular retinal detachment reached its maximum severity 80 (median) days after the renal artery clamping, and at this stage the severity of the detachment in the two eyes of an animal was unequal in about half of the animals. At the last examination, the detachment had resolved completely in about half of the animals. The subretinal fluid varied from clear (fig. 5–7] to proteinaceous or gelatinous (fig. 2–4, 8) – in some it was clear at first and later became proteinaceous, or opaque exudative type in the foveal region but clear around that, and rarely there was even subretinal hemorrhage; some eyes later developed subretinal fibrosis in the macular region (fig. 10). In a

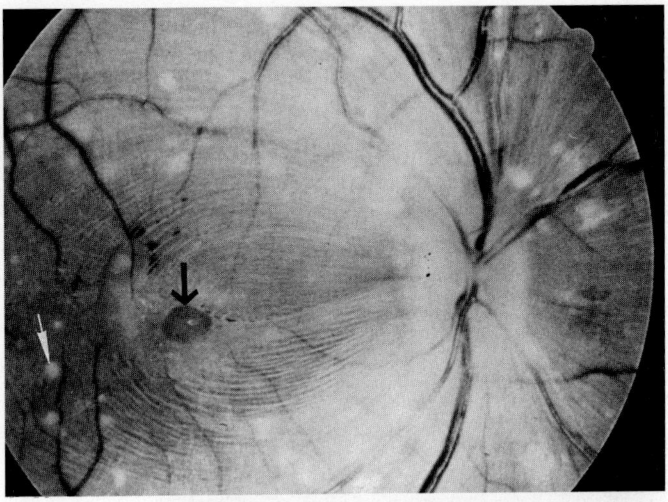

a

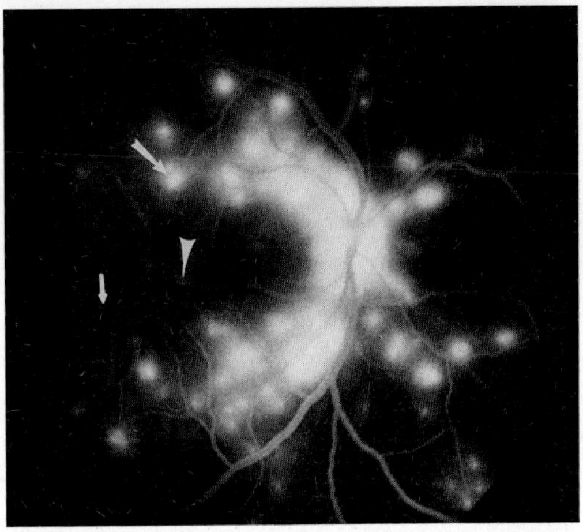

b

Fig. 6. Right eye of a monkey with BP 190 mm Hg on day 84. **a** Fundus photograph showing serous macular retinal detachment of macular region with clear subretinal fluid, macular edema with microcystic change, foveal cyst (black arrow) and separation of nerve fibers by edema, and multiple focal degenerative RPE lesions (white arrow). Published courtesy of *Ophthalmology* 1986;93:1383–1400 [3a]. **b** Fluorescein angiogram during the late phase showing multiple bright fluorescent spots due to leakage of the dye in the FIPTs (large arrow), a few faint fluorescent spots in the temporal part of the macula corresponding to the focal degenerative RPE lesions (small arrow), and faint staining of the foveal cyst (arrow head).

number of these eyes the subretinal exudative material in the macular region resolved at first in small spots, giving it a honeycomb or lacunar appearance which mimicked CME on ophthalmoscopy.

In the two-kidney model, only 4 monkeys developed the macular serous retinal detachment, first seen 52 (median) days after renal artery clamping when the median BP was 174 mm Hg. It involved both eyes in all animals. The detachment resolved in all these monkeys during follow-up.

Macular RPE Changes

These are an essential part of hypertensive choroidopathy and, as such, are discussed at length in our account of the choroidopathy [3a]. Very briefly, the RPE changes were seen

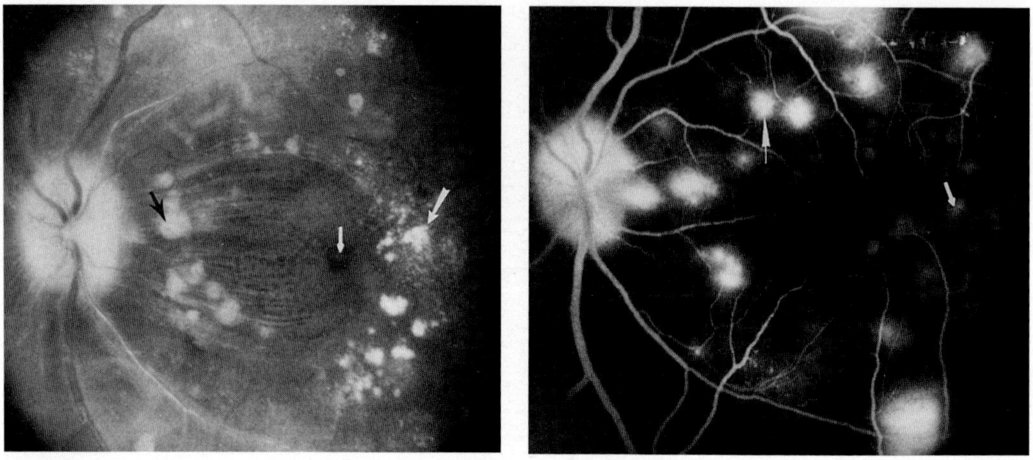

a b

Fig. 7. Left eye of a monkey with BP 212 mm Hg on day 174. **a** Fundus photograph showing serous macular retinal detachment with clear subretinal fluid, macular edema, separation of nerve fibers by edema, microcystic edema and foveal cyst (small white arrow), CWSs (black arrow), and lipid deposits (large white arrow) in the right and upper parts of the photograph. Published courtesy of *Ophthalmology* 1986;93:1383–1400 [3a]. **b** Fluorescein angiogram during the late phase showing bright fluorescent spots (large arrow) corresponding to the FIPTs (and not the CWSs), and multiple faintly fluorescent spots (small arrow), mostly in the temporal part of the macula, due to focal degenerative RPE lesions, but no staining of the microcystic lesions and foveal cyst.

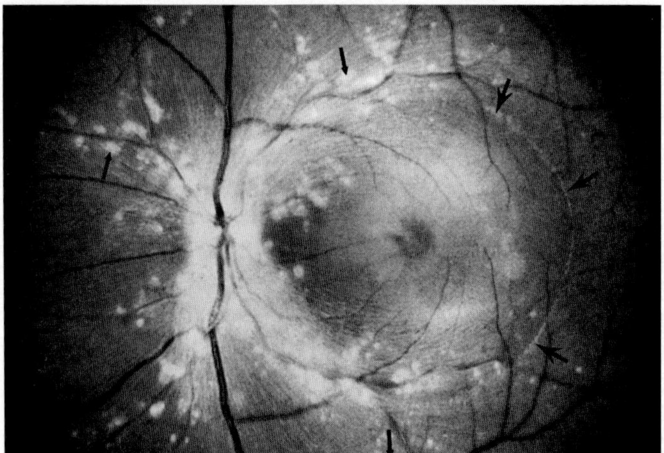

Fig. 8. Fundus photograph of left eye of a monkey with BP 204 mm Hg on day 36, showing bullous macular serous retinal detachment (large arrows) with whitish proteinaceous subretinal fluid, especially in the central part, and multiple FIPTs (small arrows). Published courtesy of *Ophthalmology* 1986;93:1383–1400 [3a].

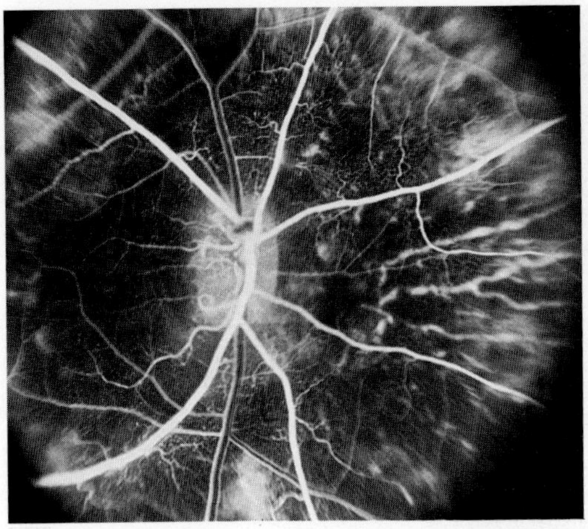

a

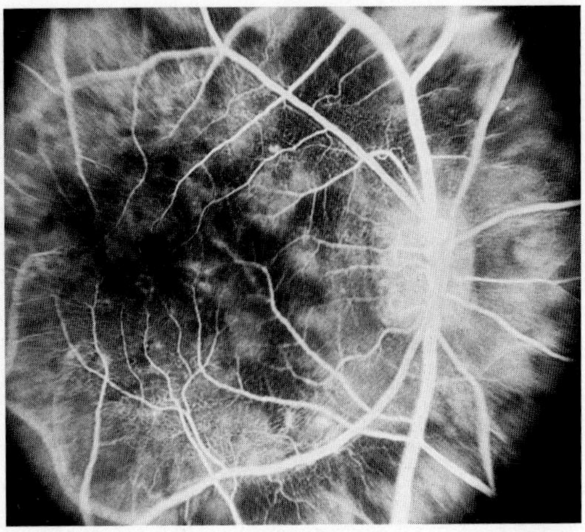

b

Fig. 9. Fluorescein fundus angiograms of right eye of a monkey with BP 170 mm Hg on day 95, showing marked choroidal filling defects during early (**a**) and late (**b**) retinal arteriovenous phases. **a** Published courtesy of *Ophthalmology* 1986;93:74 –87 [3b].

in 17 one-kidney monkeys and in 11 two-kidney monkeys at some stage of the follow-up. These RPE lesions were of two types:

Acute Focal RPE Lesions. These were first seen within 41 (median) days after the renal artery clamping, at a BP of 190 mm Hg (median) in one-kidney monkeys, and within 70 days (median), with a BP of 185 mm Hg (median) in the two-kidney model. These lesions were white or pale, punctate and round, usually located in the central and/or temporal part of the macular region (fig. 5, 6, 11a). They were generally similar in severity in the two eyes of an animal. With time these lesions gradually increased in number. Fluorescein fundus angiography almost invariably showed evidence of macular choroidal ischemia in them (fig. 9), and staining of the lesions during the late phase of angiography (fig. 5). There was an overlying serous retinal detachment in 16 of the one-kidney animals and four of the two-kidney animals, as discussed above.

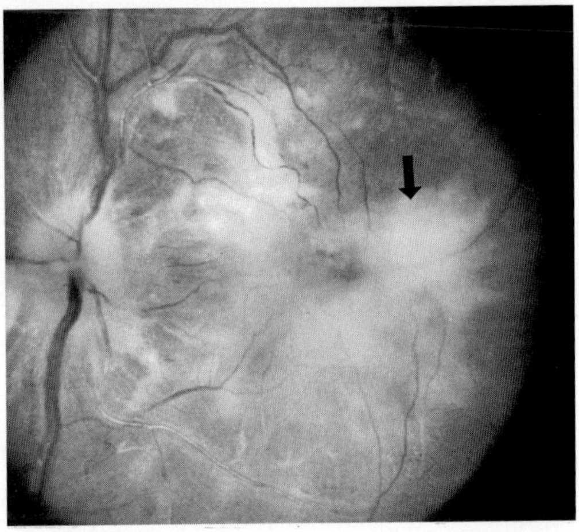

Fig. 10. Fundus photograph of left eye of a monkey with BP 250 mm Hg on day 112, showing whitish subretinal fibrosis (arrow) in the macular region. Published courtesy of *Ophthalmology* 1986;93:1383–1400 [3a].

RPE Degenerative Lesions. In 2–3 weeks the acute focal RPE lesions evolved into focal RPE degenerative lesions – depigmented focal lesions, showing on fluorescein angiography

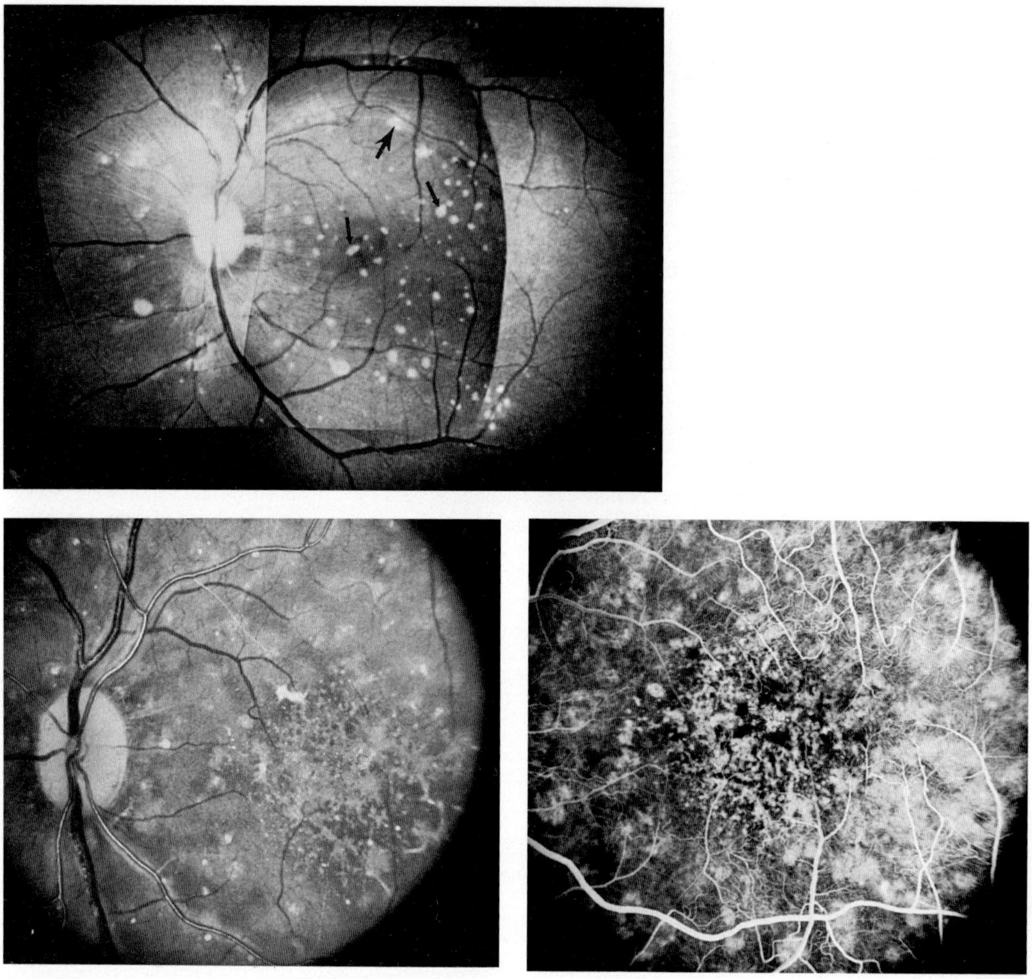

a b c

Fig. 11. Left eye of a monkey. **a** On day 41 with BP 202 mm Hg, fundus photograph showing multiple acute focal RPE lesions (small arrows), in addition to a few FIPTs (along the retinal arterioles only; large arrow) and no serous retinal detachment. **b, c** On day 354 with BP 220 mm Hg. **b** Fundus photograph showing extensive late macular RPE degenerative lesions, multiple drusen (white glistening dots) and retinal arteriolar sclerosis. **c** Fluorescein angiogram during the late retinal arteriovenous phase showing diffuse RPE degeneration in the macular region and focal RPE degeneration elsewhere.

unmasking of the underlying choroidal fluorescence of the lesions, with no late staining (fig. 3b, 6b, 7b, 11c, 12b). The degenerative lesions were almost always progressive in nature and reached their maximum within 231 days (median) after the renal artery clamping, with a BP of 195-hmm Hg (median) in one-kidney monkeys, and within 123 days (median) at 188 mm Hg (median) BP in the two-kidney model. The degenerative lesions, having

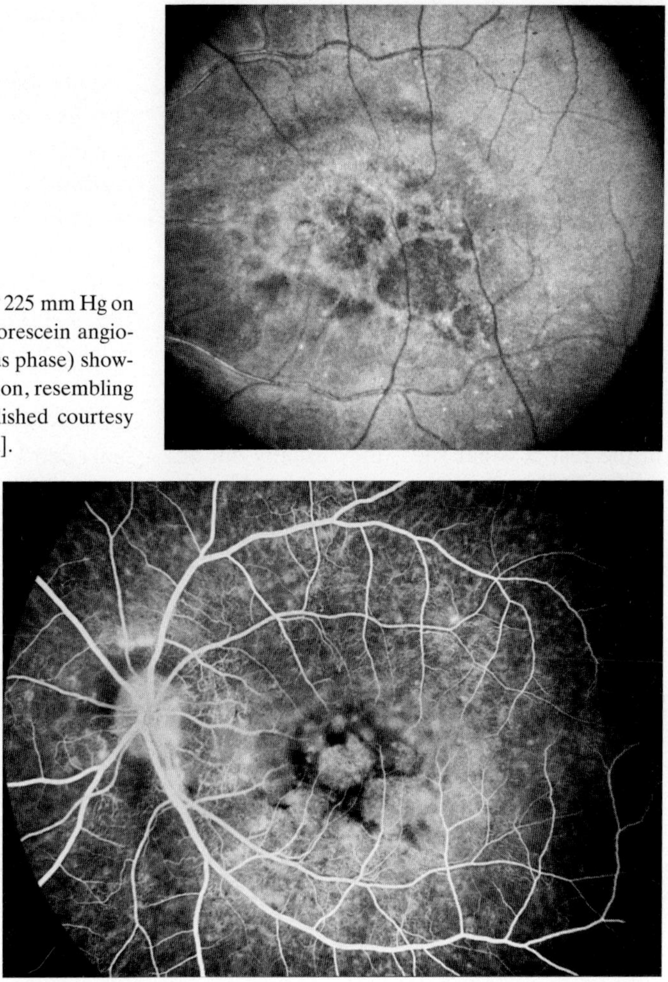

Fig. 12. Left eye of a monkey with BP 225 mm Hg on day 598. Fundus photograph (**a**) and fluorescein angiogram (**b**; during late retinal arteriovenous phase) showing RPE degeneration in the macular region, resembling age-related macular degeneration. Published courtesy of *Ophthalmology* 1986;93:1383–1400 [3a].

a

b

reached a peak, remained stationary thereafter. In the macular region, the lesions were most marked in the temporal part and not infrequently also in the foveal area, with moth-eaten-looking RPE, and less frequently subretinal fibrosis, subretinal gliosis, colloid bodies, and other RPE degenerative changes (fig. 10, 11b, 12). Fluorescein fundus angiography showed unmasking of the underlying choroidal fluorescence in depigmented areas and masking in the hyperpigmented areas (fig. 11c, 12b). These ophthalmoscopic and angiographic changes very much resembled those seen in age-related macular degeneration in man.

Macular Retinal Lipid Deposits

The 'hard exudates' or retinal lipid deposits seen in the present study are discussed in detail elsewhere [4]. Very briefly, *in the one-kidney model* the lipid deposits in the macular region were seen in 9 of the 18 animals, usually bilateral, first noted 83 days (median) after the renal artery clamping when the macular retina had edema and there was macular retinal detachment; however, there was no correlation between the presence or severity of lipid deposits and the severity or extent of retinal detachment and macular edema. These deposits lasted for about 10 weeks (median). The amount varied from no more than a few fine white granules (fig. 2) to more extensive deposits (fig. 4, 7). In 8 animals the deposits were situated in the temporal part of the foveal/macular region and in the rest at other sites; they usually did not involve the central foveolar region. *In the two-kidney model,* the lipid deposits were seen in 2 of the 5 animals with macular edema, 2 and 5 weeks after the onset of macular edema, with BPs of 190 and 215 mm Hg, respectively.

The lipid deposits in the macular region assumed different shapes, including that of an open Japanese fan with its handle at the fovea, star-shaped or irregular deposits.

Other Macular Retinal Lesions

In addition to the previously described macular retinal lesions, the usual retinal lesions associated with hypertensive retinopathy, e.g., FIPTs [2], CWSs [5] and hemorrhages [6] were frequently seen. Some of the eyes (mostly of the one-kidney model) also had other lesions which included the following: (1) retinal atrophy: this was especially marked in the macular region; (2) diaphanous appearance of the retina over the retinal detachment: this was seen in about one third of the animals and was especially marked in the macular region; (3) subretinal fibrosis: this was seen in a few eyes and usually followed the resolution of subretinal exudation (fig. 10); (4) retinal folds: these were seen over retinal detachment, especially when it was extensive and bullous in nature.

Comments

Our studies showed that macular retinal changes are a common feature of fundus changes in malignant arterial hypertension. In addition to the usual retinal lesions seen in hypertensive retinopathy associated with malignant arterial hypertension, e.g., hemorrhages [6], CWSs or inner retinal ischemic spots [5] (fig. 1–4, 7), FIPTs [2] (fig. 1, 2, 5, 7], there are some lesions which usually occurred more markedly and commonly in the macular region than elsewhere and these included macular retinal edema (fig. 1–7), separation of the surface nerve fibers (usually in the retina between the fovea and disk; fig. 2–7), foveal and macular cystic retinal change (fig. 2–7), serous retinal detachment (fig. 1–8), RPE changes (fig. 5, 6, 10–12) and lipid deposits (fig. 2, 4, 7).

Pathogenesis of Macular Edema and CME

These lesions occur in a large number of ocular and systemic conditions as well as in many types of retinopathy. There is a large volume of literature containing speculation as to the pathogenesis of the macular edema and CME seen in different conditions [7]. However, there is very little definite information available on the subject. The pathogenesis of these changes is most probably not the same in all conditions. For example, macular edema and CME following cataract extraction, retinal vein occlusion and ocular hypotony, to mention only three conditions, probably have totally different mechanisms, compared with that seen in malignant arterial hypertension. Therefore, information on the pathogenesis of macular edema and CME in one disease is not necessarily relevant to similar changes of another etiology. For instance, Yanoff et al. [8], based on light and electron microscopic examination of 2 eyes with CME associated with choroidal malignant melanoma, concluded that 'intracytoplasmic swelling (edema) of the Müller (glial) cells is the anatomical basis for the macular edema'. According to them, 'intercellular (extracellular) collections of fluid probably are late, end stage results of the proces that results from prolonged, excessive, intracellular edema, cell death and disruption'; however, they did find retinal microvascular changes as well. By contrast, Tso [9], based on his experimental studies, reviewed the subject of the pathogenesis of CME as seen in a variety of conditions. He postulated that presumably there were four sets of causative factors in the production of CME studied by him and these included: (1) disruption of the blood-retinal barrier in the retinal vasculature and the RPE; (2) ischemic retinal tissue damage with cyst formation; (3) intraocular events, e.g., inflammation, ocular hypotony, and vitreous traction, and (4) the probable additive effect on the macula of systemic diseases. He concluded that CME is the final common pathway of a multifactorial syndrome.

In the literature, unfortunately, there is very little information on the macular edema and CME seen in malignant arterial hypertension. It is the prevailing impression that macular edema and associated changes in malignant hypertension are due to microangiopathy of the retinal vascular bed. Gass [10] stated that there were no ophthalmoscopic or angiographic changes in the macular RPE in most hypertensive patients with loss of central vision, and felt that that was evidence that choroidal vascular insufficiency was probably unimportant in the pathogenesis of macular dysfunction. He further added that, even in severe hypertension with evidence of choroidal vascular involvement, the ophthalmoscopic changes in the choroidal blood vessel and overlying RPE were least evident in the posterior pole. Our experience contradicts Gass' [10] views. As discussed below, and illustrated in detail in our publication on hypertensive choroidopathy [3a], our ophthalmoscopic, fluorescein angiographic, morphologic and horseradish peroxidase studies gave irrefutable evidence that these macular changes are essentially a manifestation of hypertensive choroidopathy, and that there are marked RPE changes in the macular region in these eyes. In some eyes, however, there may be additional retinal vascular changes causing macular edema and secondary RPE changes.

Retinal edema is a well-known feature of hypertensive retinopathy. In the present study it was most pronounced in the macular region. The pathogenesis of retinal/macular edema in malignant arterial hypertension is still uncertain; it seems to be multifactorial in origin, and the following elements have been postulated for its development.

Exudative Phenomenon. Serofibrinous exudates are similar to the histopathologically seen insudation of fibrin-rich plasma within the wall of arterioles and capillaries [11, 15], seen far more frequently in microscopical than in ophthalmoscopic or fluorescein angiographic examination, probably because of the small quantities of fluid accumulation in the retinal tissue. Ashton [12], Garner [13] and Garner et al. [14] stated that generalized retinal edema can be due to autoregulatory failure, resulting in a rise in transmural pressure in distal arterioles and proximal capillaries, that permits increased transudation of fluid into the retinal tissue. It is not clear whether leakage is due to altered endothelial permeability from some unidentified circulatory factor or from an increased filtration pressure [16]. Our inability to demonstrate leakage of dye from retinal vessels on fluorescein fundus angiography in the macular region in all eyes with macular edema may have been due to insensitivity of fluorescein angiography to show such a leakage. Tso and Shih [17], in their studies on experimental postcataract extraction macular edema in monkeys, showed that in spite of the obvious disruption of blood-retinal barrier on light and electron microscopy by a horseradish peroxidase tracer technique, no such disruption was seen by fluorescein fundus angiography.

Ischemic in Nature. Ultrastructural changes seen by Garner and coworkers [12–14] indicated that intracellular edema of ischemic origin is also of importance in the production of retinal edema in malignant arterial hypertension.

Secondary to Serous Retinal Detachment. In the present study, we found an important relationship between macular edema and serous retinal detachment. In the one-kidney model, when macular edema appeared initially, almost all eyes had associated serous retinal detachment in the macular region (fig. 1–8), and the majority also had peripapillary serous retinal detachment. In two thirds of these animals, the onset of serous macular retinal detachment and of macular edema occurred almost simultaneously, while in the remainder the retinal detachment developed first. When macular edema was at its peak in this group, all the eyes had variable degrees of retinal detachment in the macular region; however, a few eyes without macular edema also had retinal detachment. In eyes where macular edema resolved during follow-up, it usually resolved before the retinal detachment, and the two rarely resolved simultaneously; however, the eyes were not examined frequently enough for definite conclusions about this relationship. In the two-kidney model also, the onset of serous retinal detachment and macular retinal edema occurred almost simultaneously.

In our previous study on hypertensive choroidopathy [3a, 18], we demonstrated that ischemic damage to the RPE plays an essential role in the development of serous retinal detachment in malignant hypertension, and we discussed the subject at length [3a]. The speculation that retinal detachment in malignant hypertension and toxemia of pregnancy is secondary to retinal changes [19–21] has no basis; moreover, retinal detachment in the complete absence of any retinopathy has been reported in the literature [22–24] and seen in this study. In this connection, it is important to note that in all the animals in this series, the development of foveal/macular edema was related to RPE infarcts. Rarely, macular edema developed without demonstrable retinal detachment, and it is probable that in these eyes, because of ischemic damage to the RPE, the fluid leaked from the choroid and seeped into the overlying retina to produce edema without an ophthalmoscopically demonstrable retinal detachment. Also, on stereoscopic examination of the color fundus photographs, the earliest evidence of macular edema was noticed in the deepest layer of the retina, suggesting a seepage of fluid from beneath. Naturally, the question arises: how can serous retinal detachment or ischemic decompensation of the RPE produce edema of the overlying retina? Since there are no barriers or tight cell junctions in the retinal tissue (unlike those in the RPE or in the retinal blood vessels) to prevent the seepage of the fluid from the subretinal space into the retinal tissue, the retina acts like a sponge and the subretinal fluid can easily move through the retinal tissue and accumulate in it. Our horseradish peroxidase studies, reported previously [3a], give evidence of this mechanism. It could be objected that in man, in eyes with routine serous retinal detachment, there is usually no apparent retinal edema on ophthalmoscopy. However, histopathologic studies in human eyes with retinal detachment have shown cystic changes and also degeneration of rods and cones if the detachment has lasted for about 4–6 weeks, and the retina tends to become edematous and atrophic, particularly in the outer layers [25]. In a few of the eyes of the present study with serous retinal detachment and no ophthalmoscopically evident retinal edema, it is possible that the edema was too subtle to be seen on ophthalmoscopy. Moreover, in the present study, we have shown the presence of definite macular edema and CME ophthalmoscopically (fig. 1–7], but these did not stain with fluorescein on fluorescein angiography and did not show a pattern of CME angiographically (fig. 3b, c, 4b, 7b); this would further support the concept that the fluid may be extremely slowly seeping from the choroid rather than from the retinal vessels.

From this discussion, it seems that macular and retinal edema may be due to one or more of the factors discussed above, acting individually or collectively.

We have discussed the subjects of pathogeneses of choroidal ischemia and secondary RPE lesions [3a] and of lipid deposits or so-called 'hard exudates' [4] elsewhere.

Conclusion

Thus, this study has revealed that, contrary to the classical textbook descriptions, in malignant arterial hypertension the macular region develops a number of lesions in the retina, RPE and choroid. These collectively constitute an important component of hypertensive fundus changes in malignant arterial hypertension and may be important in the long-term visual outcome in these patients.

Acknowledgments

We are grateful to Dr. Robert F. Woolson and Dr. Marie R. Klugman of the Department of Preventive Medicine (Biostatistics) for their help with the statistical analyses of the data, to Mrs. Ellen Ballas and Mrs. Georgiane Parkes-Perret for their secretarial help, to Mr. James Swaner for the technical help, and to the Photography Department for the illustrations. This investigation was supported by a research grant from the National Eye Institute (EY-1576) and in part by an unrestricted grant from Research to Prevent Blindness, Inc., and from Alcon Research Institute.

References

1 Hayreh SS, Servais GE, Virdi PS, et al: Fundus lesions in malignant hypertension. III. Arterial blood pressure, biochemical and fundus changes. Ophthalmology 1986;93:45–59.

2 Hayreh SS, Servais GE, Virdi PS: Fundus lesions in malignant hypertension. IV. Focal intra-retinal periarteriolar transudates. Ophthalmology 1986;93:60–73.

3a Hayreh SS, Servais GE, Virdi PS: Fundus lesions in malignant hypertension. VI. Hypertensive choroidopathy. Ophthalmology 1986;93:1383–1400.

3b Hayreh SS, Servais GE, Virdi PS: Fundus lesions in malignant hypertension. V. Hypertensive optic neuropathy. Ophthalmology 1986;93:74–87.

4 Hayreh SS, Servais, GE, Virdi PS: Retinal lipid deposits in malignant arterial hypertension. Ophthalmologica 1989;198:216–229.

5 Hayreh SS, Servais GE, Virdi PS: Cotton-wool spots (Inner retinal ischemic spots) in malignant arterial hypertension. Ophthalmologica 1989;198:197–215.

6 Hayreh SS, Servais GE: Retinal hemorrhages in malignant arterial hypertension. Int Ophthalmol 1988;12:137–145, 197.

7 Henkind P (ed): First International Cystoid Macular Edema Symp. Surv Ophthalmol 1984;28(suppl):431–619.

8 Yanoff M, Fine BS, Brucker AJ, et al: Pathology of human cystoid macular edema. Surv Ophthalmol 1984;28(suppl):505–511.

9 Tso MOM: Animal modeling of cystoid macular edema. Surv Ophthalmol 1984;28 (suppl):512–519.

10 Gass JDM: A fluorescein angiographic study of macular dysfunction secondary to retinal vascular disease. III. Hypertensive retinopathy. Arch Ophthalmol 1968;80:569–582.
11 Giacomelli F, Wiener J, Spiro D: The cellular pathology of experimental hypertension. V. Increased permeability of cerebral arterial vessels. Am J Pathol 1970;59:133–159.
12 Ashton N: The eye in malignant hypertension. Trans Am Acad Ophthalmol Otolaryngol 1972;76:17–40.
13 Garner A: Experimental Hypertensive Retinopathy; PhD thesis, London, 1972.
14 Garner A, Ashton N, Tripathi R, et al: Pathogenesis of hypertensive retinopathy: An experimental study in the monkey. Br J Ophthalmol 1975;59:3–44.
15 Oka Y, Nomura T, Nakamura M, et al: Ophthalmological studies on perinephritis hypertension in monkeys: pathogenesis of retinal changes. Nippon Ganka Gakkai Zasshi 1975;79:904–914.
16 Meyer JS, Waltz AG, Gotoh F: Pathogenesis of cerebral vasospasm in hypertensive encephalopathy. I. Effects of acute increases in intraluminal blood pressure on pial blood flow. Neurology 1960;10:735–744.
17 Tso MOM, Shih CY: Experimental macular edema after lens extraction. Invest Ophthalmol Vis Sci 1977;16:381–392.
18 Kishi S, Tso MOM, Hayreh SS: Fundus lesions in malignant hypertension. I. A pathologic study of experimental hypertensive choroidopathy. Arch Ophthalmol 1985;103:1189–1197.
19 Kenny GS, Cerasoli JR: Color fluorescein angiography in toxemia of pregnancy. Arch Ophthalmol 1972;87:383–388.
20 Moore RF: Medical Ophthalmology, ed 2. London, Blakiston, 1925, pp 189–190.
21 Friedenwald JS: Pathogenesis of albuminuric retinitis. Contributions to the Medical Sciences in Honor of Dr. Emmanuel Libman (Libman Anniversary Volumes). New York, The International Press, 1932, Vol 2 pp 453–458.
22 Hallum AV: Changes in retinal arterioles associated with hypertensions of pregnancy. Arch Ophthalmol 1947;37:472–490.
23 Oliver M, Uchenik D: Bilateral exudative retinal detachment in eclampsia without hypertensive retinopathy. Am J Ophthalmol 1980;90:792–796.
24 McEvoy M, Runciman J, Edmonds DK, et al: Bilateral retinal detachment in association with preeclampsia. Aust NZ J Obstet Gynaecol 1981;21:246–247.
25 Apple DJ, Rabb MF: Clinicopathologic Correlation of Ocular Disease, ed 2. St Louis, Mosby, 1978, p 320.

Dr. S. S. Hayreh
Department of Ophthalmology
University of Iowa Hospitals and Clinics
Iowa City, IA 52242 (USA)

Ophthalmologica 1989;198:247–260

Classification of Hypertensive Fundus Changes and Their Order of Appearance

Sohan Singh Hayreh

Department of Ophthalmology, University of Iowa, Iowa City, Iowa, USA

Key Words. Arterial hypertension · Classification · Fundus lesions · Hypertensive retinopathy · Malignant arterial hypertension · Order of appearance · Retinal lesions

Abstract. We studied the sequence of appearance of the various fundus lesions in experimentally produced renovascular malignant arterial hypertension in 60 rhesus monkeys. The earliest lesion to appear usually was focal intraretinal periarteriolar transudates (FIPTs). Some time after that, three lesions: acute focal retinal pigment epithelial lesions, macular edema and optic disk edema, developed at roughly the same time. Cotton-wool spots appeared after these lesions. Retinal lipid deposits developed relatively late. Retinal arteriolar changes were a much later phenomenon. Conspicuous retinal hemorrhages were not a common or prominent early sign. The various classifications of hypertensive fundus changes proposed in the literature are reviewed and discussed critically, and it is concluded that, instead of using the various arbitrary grades advocated in different classifications, it is more informative and clinically useful to give a descriptive account of the individual fundus lesions revealed by ophthalmoscopy and fluorescein fundus angiography; because different lesions have different degrees of significance.

The ophthalmologist may be the first physician whom a patient with malignant arterial hypertension consults; he/she may come with visual disturbance directly attributable to malignant hypertension, or the ophthalmologist may observe hypertensive fundus changes though they are unrelated to the patient's original complaint. Under such circumstances, the ophthalmologist will wish to know about the duration and severity of both malignant hypertension and the fundus changes secondary to it. Frequently, the only guide to this has been the so-called 'grade of hypertensive retinopathy'. Since 1939, multiple classifications and methods of grading of hypertensive fundus changes have been put forward [1–6]. All were based on ophthalmoscopic interpretation of the fundus changes, particularly retinal arteriolar changes. With the advent of fluorescein fundus angiography and a better understanding of the pathophysiology of the various fundus lesions in malignant arterial hypertension, the limitations of these various schemes have become apparent.

In our studies on experimental renovascular malignant arterial hypertension in rhesus monkeys, ophthalmoscopic, fluorescein fundus angiographic and pathologic studies clearly showed that the various fundus changes fall into three distinct categories [7–12]: (1) hypertensive retinopathy, (2) hypertensive choroidopathy [8, 12], and (3) hypertensive optic neuropathy [7, 11]. Unfortunately, in the past, all the fundus changes in malignant hypertension have been mistakenly categorized as 'hypertensive retinopathy'. In our studies, we reported that hypertensive retinopathy appeared significantly ($p<0.01$) earlier than hypertensive choroidopathy or optic neuropathy [9]. Our studies also revealed that in monkeys of the one-kidney one-clip model, the rise in blood pressure (BP) developed significantly ($p=0.01$) faster and the fundus lesions appeared significantly ($p=0.00001$) earlier than in the two-kidney one-clip model [9].

In view of these various considerations, we investigated the sequence of appearance of the various early, major fundus lesions in malignant arterial hypertension in the one-kidney model, and then critically reviewed and evaluated the relevance of different classifications and gradings in the light of our current knowledge on the subject.

Material and Methods

This study is based on findings in 60 rhesus monkeys in which experimental renovascular malignant arterial hypertension was produced by modified Goldblatt's procedures. The methods used in this study are described in detail elsewhere [9]. Briefly, the animals consisted of two groups: *one-kidney one-clip model* (25 monkeys) which had nephrectomy on one side and the remaining kidney was made ischemic by a renal clamp, and *two-kidney one-clip model* (35 monkeys) that had both kidneys – one normal but the other made ischemic with a renal clamp. The animals were investigated by recording BP, ophthalmoscopy (direct and indirect), stereoscopic color fundus photography and fluorescein fundus angiography before renal artery clamping and serially thereafter. Our method of BP recording gave reliable information only on the systolic BP [9].

Data Analyses

The BP, ophthalmoscopic and fluorescein angiographic findings in the animals were critically reviewed and tabulated for each animal for every examination conducted during the longitudinal follow-up; this had to be customized for each animal, because of the delicate health of the animals during severe malignant hypertension, the hazards of nembutal general anesthesia required for each fundus examination, and the logistic problems of carrying out these time-consuming procedures. The data from the two models were finally collated and analyzed separately. The median (50th percentage point in data) and interquartile range (IQR; the difference between the 25th and 75th percentage points) were calculated for most of the parameters because these statistics give a much better picture of the center and spread of a distribution than do the mean and standard deviation in data with extreme values, which was frequently the case in the present study. Statistical significances were calculated by using the Wilcoxon rank sum test and the Spearman correlation coefficient.

Results

BP, Hypertensive Retinopathy, Choroidopathy and Optic Neuropathy, and Follow-Up Period

Table 1 summarizes the data on the BP, incidence of hypertensive retinopathy, choroidopathy and optic neuropathy, and length of follow-up. The general BP changes in this experimental study are discussed at length elsewhere [9]. In normal adult rhesus monkeys the normal median systolic BP was 120 (with IQR 15) mm Hg. As judged from BP levels seen in human arterial hypertension, we decided to consider a systolic BP of ≥160 mm Hg as hy-

Table 1. Length of follow-up, BP findings and hypertensive retinopathy in one-kidney and two-kidney animals

	One-kidney group (25 monkeys)			Two-kidney group (35 monkeys)		
	range	median	IQR	range	median	IQR
Follow-up period, months	1.2–57.3[1]	9.6[1]	19.2[1]	0.7–42.3	26.4	10.5
Time interval (days) from renal artery clamping to						
Onset of hypertension	2– 43	7	3	2–115	15	18
Maximum BP recorded	2–980	110	287	8–899	124	237
Onset of hypertensive retinopathy	12– 63[2]	22[2]	17[2]	8–302[3]	64[3]	44[3]
Onset of hypertensive choroidopathy	15–133[2]	41[2]	27[2]	15–284[4]	71.5[4]	69[4]
Onset of hypertensive Optic neuropathy	16–168[2]	37[2]	33[2]	20–135[5]	35[5]	86[5]
Highest BP recorded						
BP level, in mm Hg	178–260	220	30	160–260	204	50
% Rise from baseline BP	148–245	193	46	133–237	175	26
BP (mmHg) at onset of						
Hypertensive retinopathy	164–225[2]	190[2]	21[2]	160–210[3]	178[3]	26[3]
Hypertensive choroidopathy	160–240[2]	190[2]	20[2]	160–230[4]	180[4]	30[4]
Hypertensive optic neuropathy	164–238[2]	190[2]	21[2]	160–214[5]	188[5]	27[5]

1 In 20 animals that survived ≥3 weeks.
2 Hypertensive retinopathy and choroidopathy both seen in 19 one-kidney monkeys.
3 Hypertensive retinopathy seen in 19 two-kidney monkeys.
4 Hypertensive choroidopathy seen in 14 two-kidney monkeys.
5 Hypertensive optic neuropathy seen in 8 two-kidney monkeys.

pertensive. Renovascular hypertension developed in all the 60 monkeys of the present series. One-kidney monkeys developed much more rapid and more severe hypertension than the two-kidney animals. Five of the 25 one-kidney monkeys died within 3 weeks after renal artery clamping from complications of accelerated hypertension or uremia. Some evidence of hypertensive retinopathy developed in 19 one-kidney monkeys (out of the 20 surviving 3≥ weeks) and 19 two-kidney animals. One or another ophthalmoscopically visible lesion of hypertensive choroidopathy developed in 19 one-kidney and 14 two-kidney animals, while fluorescein fundus angiographic abnormalities of the choroidal vascular bed developed in 20 and 16 monkeys, respectively. Hypertensive optic neuropathy was seen in 17 of the 19 one-

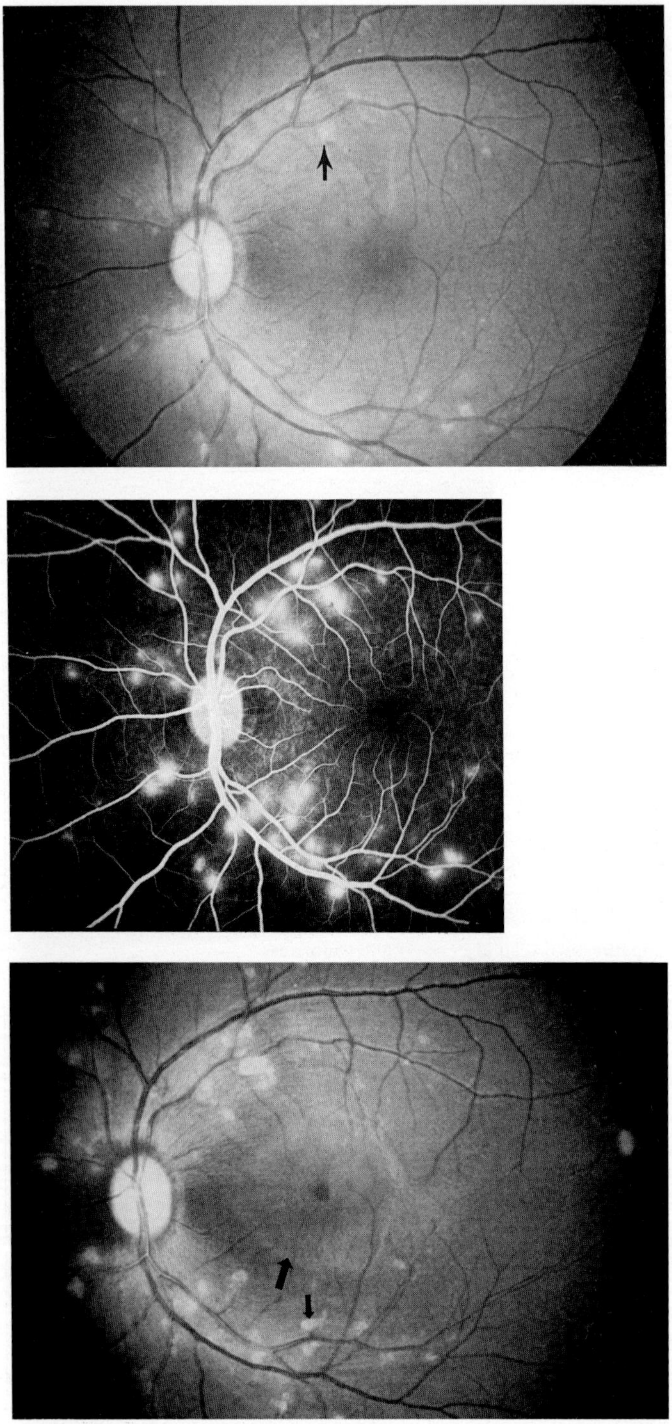

a

b

c

Fig. 1. Ophthalmoscopic (**a, c**) and fluorescein angiographic (**b**) appearance of left eye of a one-kidney monkey. **a, b** 43 days after renal artery clamping with BP 225 mm Hg. **a** Many FIPTs (arrow). **b** Focal fluorescein leakage corresponding to the FIPTs. **c** On day 50 with BP 214 mm Hg: more extensive FIPTs (small arrow) than in **a** and localized macular edema (large arrow). **a, c** Published courtesy of *Ophthalmology* 1986;93: 60–73 [10].

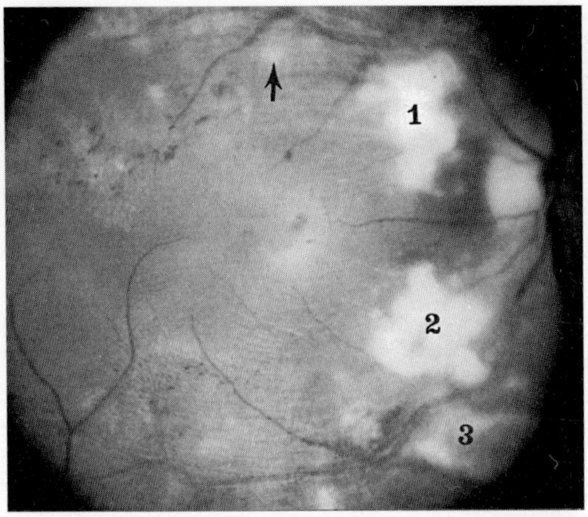

a

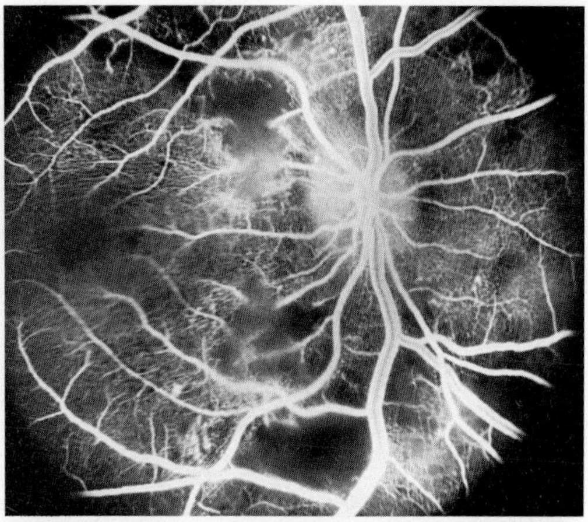

b

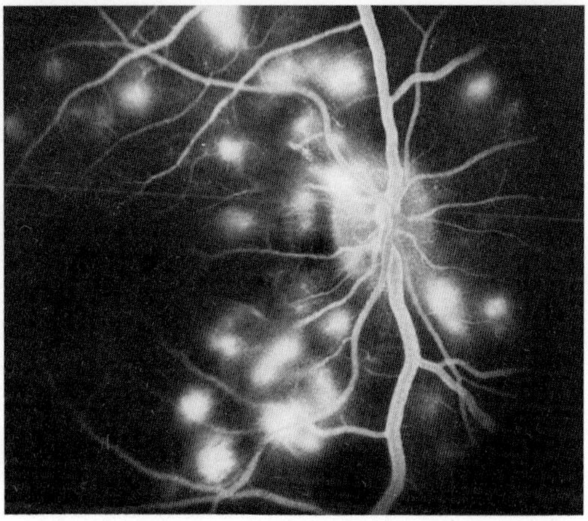

c

Fig. 2. Ophthalmoscopic (**a**) and fluorescein angiographic (**b, c**) appearance in right eye of one-kidney monkey on day 56 with BP 240 mm Hg. **a** Two fresh CWSs (No. 1 and 2), in addition to a resolving CWS (No. 3) and FIPTs (arrow), a few fine hemorrhages, marked macular edema and macular serous retinal detachment with opaque exudative subretinal fluid. **b, c** During the retinal arteriovenous phase (**b**), shows retinal capillary nonperfusion in the distribution of the fresh and resolving cotton-wool spots, and during the late phase (**c**) shows leaking spots only in the distribution of the FIPTs, and *none* in the region of the CWSs. In the region of the CWS No. 2, situated inferotemporal to the optic disk, there are some underlying FIPTs (best seen on stereoscopic examination) which are responsible for the fluorescein leakage in that area.

kidney monkeys, and in 8 of the two-kidney monkeys.

Order of Appearance of the Various Early, Major Fundus Lesions of Malignant Arterial Hypertension in the One-Kidney Model

Early, Major Retinal Lesions in Hypertensive Retinopathy. Figures 1–4 illustrate most of the retinal lesions seen in hypertensive retinopathy. We investigated the sequence of appearance of the first six retinal lesions in the one-kidney model, which provided the major part of the information on the subject. Table 2 summarizes the findings on the order of appearance, the time after the renal artery clamping and the BP at which the first six retinal lesions developed. Some of the animals, in spite of long survival, never developed more than two or three lesions.

Days of onset of all the six types of lesions in table 2 showed significant ($p \leq 0.01$) correla-

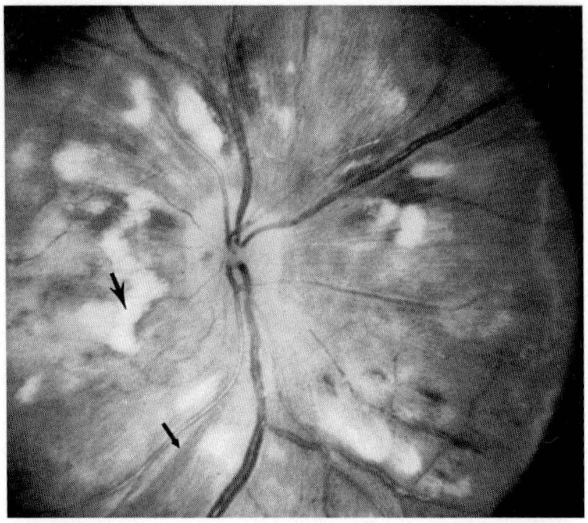
a

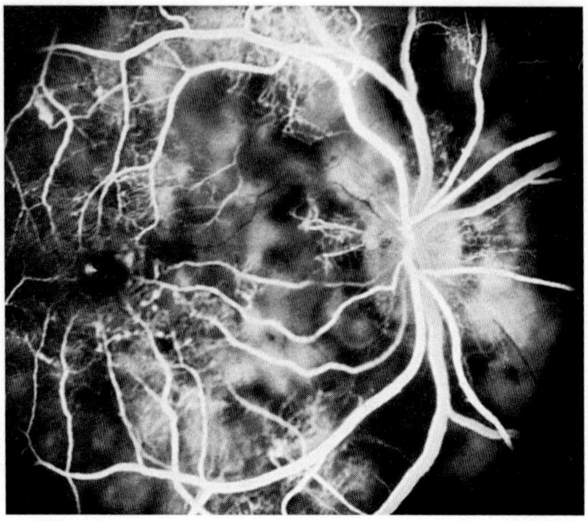
b

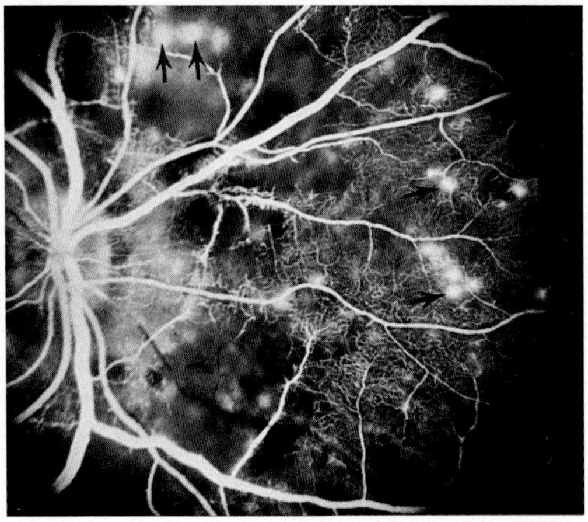
c

Fig. 3. Ophthalmoscopic (**a**) and fluorescein angiographic (**b, c**) appearance of right eye of a one-kidney monkey on day 126 with BP 214 mm Hg. **a** Shows multiple CWSs (large arrow), retinal hemorrhages, nerve fiber loss (small arrow), and arteriolar sclerosis. **b, c** Show retinal capillary nonperfusion in the distribution of the CWSs seen in **a** as well as in those which developed in the past but had resolved by this time; fluorescein leaking spots (arrows) in **c** represent FIPTs. **c** Published courtesy of *Ophthalmology* 1986;93:60–73 [10].

tions with each other except between the first two lesions. Similarly, BP levels between the first three types of lesions showed significant ($p \leq 0.03$) correlations.

Early, Major Fundus Lesions in Hypertension. We recorded the time interval between the Goldblatt's procedure and the first appearance of the early, major fundus lesions, and the BP at those times. The data are given in table 3. I want to stress that, unlike these important major lesions, retinal hemorrhages were usually minor, inconspicuous fundus lesions, mostly only one or two in number early on, and some of them might be merely fortuitous in nature. Therefore they are not included in table 3.

In the two-kidney model, in view of the slow development of hypertension and of various fundus lesions, the marked variability in the data, and the less distinct pattern than was seen in one-kidney model, we could not do a similar analysis. It would not have yielded any useful information on the subject.

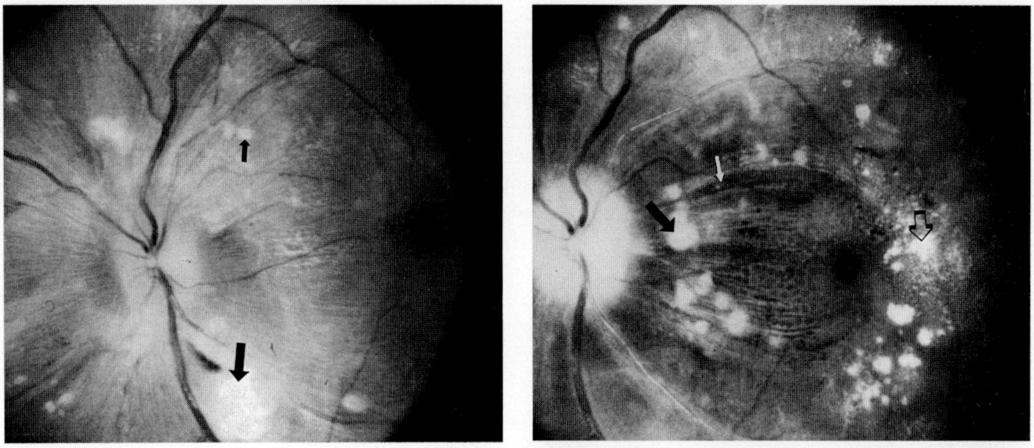

a b

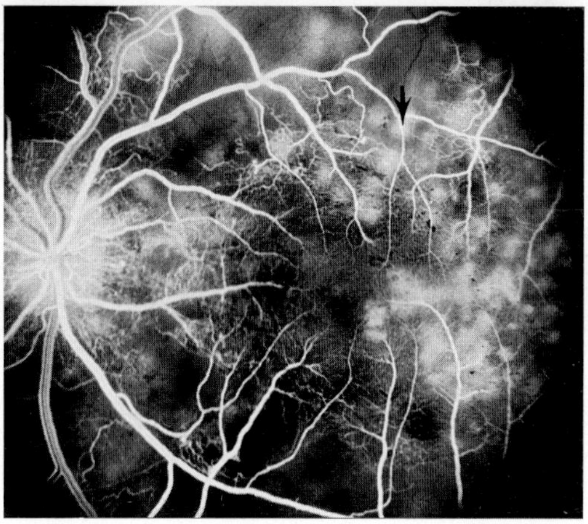

c

Fig. 4. Ophthalmoscopic (**a, b**) and fluorescein angiographic (**c**) appearance of a one-kidney monkey. **a** On day 63 with BP 192 mm Hg, shows a CWS (large arrow), multiple FIPTs (small arrow) and a hemorrhage. **b, c** On day 174 with BP 212 mm Hg. **b** CWSs (large arrow), microcystic macular edema, nerve fiber loss (small white arrow), lipid deposits (hollow arrow), and arteriolar sclerosis. **c** Extensive retinal capillary nonperfusion in the distribution of previously seen CWSs. Fluorescent spots (arrow) seen in the temporal and superior part of the macular region are due to focal retinal pigment epithelial lesions which are one of the lesions of hypertensive choroidopathy. **a, b** are Published courtesy of *Ophthalmology* 1986;93:60–73, 1383–1400 [10, 12], respectively.

Comments

Various Early, Major Fundus Lesions of Malignant Arterial Hypertension and Their Sequence of Appearance

Early, Major Retinal Lesions of Hypertensive Retinopathy. It is generally believed in clinical ophthalmology and is stressed in the literature that retinal hemorrhages are an important early manifestation of hypertensive retinopathy due to malignant arterial hypertension [13–16]. Also cotton-wool spots (CWSs), retinal edema, lipid deposits and retinal arteriolar changes have been long described as the classical early findings in hypertensive retinopathy. However, there is hardly any information on the sequence of appearance of these retinal lesions and their importance in evaluation of severity and duration of arterial hypertension. Moreover, there is a fair amount of misinformation prevalent about the various lesions seen in hypertensive retinopa-

Table 2. Sequence of appearance of the first six retinal lesions of hypertensive retinopathy in the 19 animals of the one-kidney model which developed hypertensive retinopathy

	Order of appearance of various retinal lesions, number of animals					
	first lesion	second lesion	third lesion	fourth lesion	fifth lesion	sixth lesion
Types of retinal lesion						
FIPTs [10]	16	3	0	0	0	0
Macular edema/CME	1	9	4	2	0	0
CWS	1	7	6	3	0	0
Retinal hemorrhages	1	0	5	2	0	0
Lipid deposits	0	0	1	3	4	1
Nerve fiber loss	0	0	1	2	1	3
Arteriolar changes	0	0	0	2	4	2
Venous changes	0	0	0	1	1	1
None	0	0	2	3	6	8
Time of development, days						
Range	12–54	16–112	16–203	19–334	21–168	22–188
Median (IQR)	25 (6)	39 (43)	50 (41)	73.5 (40)	77 (56)	104 (59)
Systolic BP, mm Hg						
Range	160–225	160–238	160–240	160–240	160–240	178–240
Median (IQR)	190 (42)	190 (29)	190 (36)	190 (32)	190 (8)	198 (20)

CME = Cystoid macular edema.

Table 3. Time of the first appearance of early major fundus lesions in one-kidney model: time interval since Goldblatt's procedure and BP at that time

Fundus lesions	Time interval, days			Blood pressure mm Hg		
	range	median	IQR	range	median	IQR
FIPTs	12– 97	27	14	160–225	190	21
Acute focal RPE lesions	16–203	34	27	160–238	188	28
Macular edema/CME	16–168	36	54	160–238	190	25
Optic disk edema	16–168	37	33	164–238	190	21
CWSs	19–203	49.5	35	178–240	199	25
Lipid deposits	22–168	69.5	34	173–240	191	24
Retinal arteriolar changes	29–407	97	57	190–240	210	18

CME = Cystoid macular edema; RPE = retinal pigment epithelial.

thy, because lesions which represent hypertensive choroidopathy [12] and optic neuropathy [11] have erroneously been believed to be parts of hypertensive retinopathy. Not only that, but there is also a good deal of confusion on the nature of the various retinal lesions. For example, focal intraretinal periarteriolar transudates (FIPTs) [10] (fig. 1, 2, 3c, 4a) have been erroneously considered to be either CWSs (fig. 2–4) or their precursors [17]. Retinal arteriolar 'spasm' has been described in the literature as a diagnostic and classical lesion of hypertensive retinopathy due to malignant hypertension – yet we found no trace of it [18].

In our studies (table 2), with accelerated rise in BP, the first retinal lesion to appear was usually the FIPT [10] (fig. 1, 2, 3c, 4a). The second lesion was usually macular edema (fig. 1c, 2a), followed by CWSs (fig. 2–4). This sequence of appearance is also indicated by table 3. A conspicuous retinal hemorrhage appeared infrequently (fig. 3a), but did not constitute an important early finding in this study in the vast majority of the animals [19] – this conflicts with the prevalent impression in the ophthalmic community [13–16]. The other retinal lesions, e.g., lipid deposits (fig. 4b), cystoid macular changes (fig. 4b), retinal arteriolar changes (fig. 3a, 4b) and nerve fiber loss (fig. 3a, 4b), developed later in the course of the disease and did not constitute early lesions of hypertensive retinopathy in malignant hypertension.

Early, Major Fundus Lesions. Table 3 shows that the order of development of the various early, major fundus lesions was as follows:

(1) the earliest lesion to develop was almost always FIPTs [10];

(2) the next three lesions, some time later, developed at roughly the same time and were the acute focal RPE lesions, macular edema/cystoid macular edema and optic disk edema.

(3) the subsequent lesion was usually CWSs;

(4) Relatively late lesions: retinal lipid deposits appeared relatively late; retinal arteriolar changes developed even much later, after arterial hypertension had lasted for some time.

Thus, in *conclusion,* our studies showed that usually the FIPT is the earliest sign of recent accelerated arterial hypertension (fig. 1a), and acute focal retinal pigment epithelial lesions, macular edema (fig. 1c, 2a) and optic disk edema are other early signs of malignant arterial hypertension, followed later by CWSs (fig. 2, 4a). Marked retinal hemorrhages are not usually an early sign of hypertensive retinopathy (fig. 1, 2a, 4a). Lipid deposits, when present, develop late, and the retinal arteriolar changes much later still.

Classification of Hypertensive Fundus Changes

In order to place the various classifications put forward during the past half a century and constantly perpetuated, in true perspective, it is absolutely essential to review and discuss them critically. The first and most widely used classification has been that of Keith et al. [1]. They graded 'hypertensive retinopathy' cases into four groups 'from the prognostic standpoint' (with very serious prognosis for groups 3 and 4 as compared to groups 1 and 2). This grading was based on histologic findings in the arterioles of pectoralis muscle biopsy and follow-up information. The authors described the following criteria for the grading:

Group 1 (benign hypertension): had few anatomic changes in the arterioles of muscles and had a good prognosis; the retinal arterioles showed 'only mild narrowing (increased tonus) or sclerosis'.

Group 2 (more marked hypertension without retinopathy): had a higher and more sustained hypertension than group 1, no retinopathy but had 'moderate to marked sclerosis of the retinal arterioles' and might show retinal vein thrombosis or arteriosclerosis, more frequent arteriolar changes in muscle, and patients may live for many years.

Group 3 (mild 'angiospastic' retinopathy): often had high and sustained hypertension and thickened arterioles, 'angiospastic' retinopathy ('edema, cotton-wool patches, and hemorrhages in the retina superimposed on a combination of sclerotic and spastic lesions in the arterioles'), more marked and numerous changes in muscle arterioles than in group 1, and high mortality.

Group 4 (malignant hypertension): 79% of the patients in this group died within 1 year, and they had persistent high BP, diffuse peripheral arterial thickening, 'angiospastic retinopathy' like that seen in group 3, with an additional 'measurable edema of the disks', and finally failure of functions of the brain, heart and kidney simultaneously.

The majority of those cases belonged to group 1, a moderate number to group 2, and only a few to group 3.

This classification by Keith et al. [1] has multiple limitations and these include the following:

(1) A disease process should be described progressively, i.e. stage 1 leading to 2, then to 3 and finally stage 4; but this is not true of this classification. For example, stages 3 and 4 are not always progressive stages of 1 and 2.

(2) This classification does not distinguish adequately the hypertensive and arteriolar sclerotic components of the vascular changes; the features of hypertensive change are CWSs, lipid deposits, increased vascular permeability and other lesions, while those of arteriolar sclerosis are arteriolar constriction and arteriovenous crossing changes.

(3) Arteriolar sclerosis due to aging can produce some of the changes recorded in this classification.

(4) Separation of the first two groups is arbitrary and depends upon the bias of an observer.

(5) Many different features may occur in each group and mix in varying degrees, resulting in heterogeneous groups.

(6) There are patients who do not fall into any of the defined categories.

(7) Our studies showed that during the acute phase of malignant hypertension there is no 'angiospastic' change of the ophthalmoscopically seen retinal arterioles [18] so that the term 'angiospastic' retinopathy has no scientific basis. Ophthalmoscopically seen narrowing of the retinal arterioles simply represents pseudo-narrowing – an ophthalmoscopic artifact [18].

(8) The criterion that the mere presence of optic disk edema denotes stage 4 is not justified. According to this classification, the great majority of patients with optic disk edema (i.e. grade 4 retinopathy) die within 1 year. These authors advocated that optic disk edema was of great prognostic significance and an ominous sign. Recently McGregor et al. [20], in 96 consecutive patients with hypertensive retinopathy and optic disk edema, on multivariate analysis, found that optic disk edema was not related to survival, and concluded that optic disk edema is an unreliable physical sign and does not adversely influence prognosis in hypertensive patients; they advocated that optic disk edema should no longer be regarded as a necessary feature of malignant hypertension! I fully agree with this view.

The clinical usefulness of this classification has been made obsolete by its many limitations, by the great advances in our knowledge of the pathophysiology of arterial hypertension and its ocular manifestations, and by the availability of highly effective antihypertensive therapy. The authors themselves admitted limitations in their classification and pointed out that 'not all cases fall into one of the four groups'.

In 1947 the American Ophthalmological Society appointed a committee (composed of Drs. Wagener, Clay and Gipner [2]) to classify hypertensive retinopathy. They suggested that different terminologies should be used for various types of hypertensive retinopathy, and these included retinopathy of: acute hypertension/chronic hypertension/terminal malignant hypertension/acute hypertension in glomerulonephritis/chronic progressive hypertension in glomerulonephritis/terminal malignant hypertension in glomerulonephritis; and they called their 'acute hypertension' also 'angioplastic hypertension'. In 'acute or angioplastic hypertension' without any arteriosclerosis, they listed the diagnostic lesions in the retina as generalized narrowing of arterioles, focal constriction of arterioles, edema of retina, CWSs, hemorrhages (usually), optic disk edema (often); according to them, these cases may terminate in recovery, in chronic hypertension, or in rapidly progressive (fulminating) malignant hypertension. This classification is of little use clinically because not only is it highly complex but also their grading of retinal arteriolar narrowing is clinically impractical; moreover, as stressed earlier, our studies revealed no 'spasm' of the ophthalmoscopically visible retinal arterioles in malignant hypertension [18] so that the term 'angioplastic hypertension' is not valid.

Scheie [3], in 1953, graded the hypertensive and arteriolar sclerotic changes separately. This classification assumed that arteriolar sclerosis is due only to hypertension and ignored the fact that it is also an aging process. Once again its grading is based on very subjective criteria and is of little clinical usefulness.

Leishman [4] in 1957 classified hypertensive retinal changes into seven highly complicated and confusing groups, once again of little practical importance.

Cogan [5] advocated his own classification, based solely on the degree of arteriolar narrowing: grade 1 with mild narrowing and grade 4 with severe narrowing. This classification elects arteriolar narrowing as the only important sign of hypertensive retinopathy, which is not valid at all. Moreover, aging change, without any associated hypertension, can also produce arteriolar narrowing. Cogan [5] himself stated that 'over-interpretation of arterial narrowing in the fundus is a common failing. When one knows the patient has hypertension, one tends to attach undue significance to questionable changes'.

Tso and Jampol [6] divided hypertensive retinopathy into (1) a vasoconstrictive phase, (2) an exudative phase, (3) a sclerotic phase, and (4) complications of the sclerotic phase. According to them, in the vasoconstrictive phase an abrupt rise of BP causes pliable and nonsclerotic retinal vessels to increase their vascular tone by autoregulation. In the exudative phase the blood-retinal barrier is disrupted, with plasma and formed blood elements leaking into the retina, particularly in the macular region. If the BP rise is not severe, there may be no exudative phase, and sclerotic changes may develop gradually, manifesting as copper-wiring or eventually silver-wiring. Complications include macroaneurysm formation, microaneurysms, central retinal artery or vein occlusion, branch vein occlusion and epiretinal membrane. Our studies have shown that the so-called vasoconstriction of the ophthalmoscopically visible retinal arterioles is not a genuine change but an ophthalmoscopic artifact [18]; the terminal retinal arterioles which may show autoregulatory vasoconstriction are too minute to be visible ophthalomoscopically. According to Leishman [4], recording of clinicial signs, such as 'copper-wiring' and 'silver-wiring' 'may become the self-imposed limit of legitimate clinical thought concerning the retinal vessels' in hypertension, and he further added that these terms have been used by most ophthalmologists without 'a clear conception of the meaning of these appearances'; thus they serve no useful purpose. Our study fully supports these ideas. Moreover, in a clinical situation, one does not find these various phases defined as separate entities, and usually the various changes are seen in different combinations in different individuals, depending upon a number of factors. Thus, once again, clinically this is not a valid classification.

All these classifications were based on purely ophthalmoscopic interpretation of the fundus changes, particularly the arteriolar changes. It is well known that such an ophthalmoscopic evaluation is not only too subjective to be of any scientific validity but also suffers from many artifacts. For example, retinal arteriolar narrowing is usually evaluated by comparing the width of a retinal arteriole with that of the accompanying retinal vein. How reliable is this observation? In 1966 the World Health Organization convened a seven member expert committee to study signs of fundus changes in arterial hypertension [21]. In 630 color transparencies of the fundus of a population sample of men aged 50, each observer evaluated this parameter. For narrowing of the retinal arterioles intraobserver disagreement was 33±12% and the interobserver disagreement was 42±17% [21]. Thus it is like tossing a coin. The unreliability of the arteriovenous ratio as a means of diagnosing arteriolar narrowing has also been stressed strongly by Stokoe and Turner [22], Evelyn et al. [23] and others. Our studies revealed that the so-called retinal arteriolar narrowing seen in hypertensive retinopathy during the initial acute phase simply represents an ophthalmoscopic artifact because of masking of a part of the arteriole by the surrounding retinal edema [18] – on fluorescein angiography the ophthalmoscopically narrow retinal arterioles showed normal lumens. Thus, based on these classifications, it is not always possible to differentiate hypertensives from nonhypertensives, let alone differentiate various severities of hypertensive disease. Malignant hypertension appears de novo in only a minority of cases; it is usually antedated by benign hypertension [24]. Therefore the retinopathy may represent a mixture of the findings of the two types of retinopathy and one may influence the findings of the other. None of these classifications took into consideration fluorescein angiographic findings, which are very important in understanding the pathophysiology of the various retinal lesions.

On ophthalmoscopy, the retinal lesions have been the most striking and evident findings in malignant arterial hypertension. This led to a firm impression in the medical profession that hypertensive retinopathy is the sole pathology in this disease in the fundus. Optic disk edema, seen in severe cases, generally has been thought to be an extension of hypertensive retinopathy. As discussed earlier, our studies [7–12] clearly showed that various fundus changes seen with malignant arterial hypertension fall into three distinct categories: (1) hypertensive retinopathy, (2) hypertensive choroidopathy [7, 12], and (3) hypertensive optic neuropathy [8, 11]. Since the blood vessels are the primary tissue to respond to an acute rise in BP, their basic properties in the retina, the choroid, and the optic nerve head determine their response to malignant hypertension. For example, *autoregulation* is present in the retinal and optic nerve head vessels but not in the choroidal vessels, *blood-tissue barrier* is present in the retinal but not in the choroidal vessels and also not in the optic nerve head, and *autonomic nerve supply* is present in the choroid but not in the retina. Because of their different anatomic and physiologic properties, the retinal and choroidal blood vessels and optic nerve head respond differently to malignant arterial hypertension; this makes hypertensive retinopathy, choroidopathy, and optic neuropathy three independent and unrelated manifestations of malignant hypertension – a fact not considered in the past in any of the classifications. Our studies revealed that hypertensive retinopathy appeared significantly ($p<0.01$) earlier than choroidopathy or optic neuropathy, and that there was no significant difference between the times of appearance of choroidopathy and optic neuropathy.

Conclusion

Thus I strongly discourage grading 'hypertensive retinopathy' but recommend giving a descriptive account of the individual fundus lesions, revealed by ophthalmoscopy and fluorescein fundus angiography. That is far more informative and useful in follow-up and estimation of severity of the hypertensive fundus changes rather than the various arbitrary grades advocated. Different hypertensive fundus lesions in a patient may have different severities, as indicated by our present study (fig. 1–4). Moreover, because of differences in pathogeneses of the various lesions in hypertensive fundus changes, different lesions have different significance. I feel that the various classifications used in the past should be stored in the museums of medicine as historic relics of our past inadequate knowledge of arterial hypertension and its management, as well as of fundus changes.

Acknowledgments

I am grateful to my wife Shelagh for her help in the preparation of this manuscript and to Mrs. Ellen Ballas and Mrs. Georgiane Parkes-Perret for their secretarial help, to Mr. James Swaner for his technical help, and to the Photography Department for the illustrations. This investigation was supported by a research grant from the National Eye Institute (EY-1576) and in part by an unrestricted grant from Research to Prevent Blindness, Inc., and from the Alcon Research Institute.

References

1 Keith NM, Wagener HP, Barker NW: Some different types of essential hypertension: Their course and prognosis. Am J Med Sci 1939;197:332–343.
2 Wagener HP, Clay GE, Gipner JF: Classification of retinal lesions in the presence of vascular hypertension. Trans Am Ophthalmol Soc 1947;45:57–73.
3 Scheie HG: Evaluation of ophthalmoscopic changes of hypertension and arteriolar sclerosis. Arch Ophthalmol 1953;49:117–138.
4 Leishman R: The eye in general vascular disease – Hypertension and arteriosclerosis. Br J Ophthalmol 1957;41:641–701.
5 Cogan DG: Ophthalmic Manifestations of Systemic Vascular Disease. Philadelphia, Saunders, 1974, pp 74–78.
6 Tso MOM, Jampol LM: Pathophysiology of hypertensive retinopathy. Ophthalmology 1982;89:1132–1145.
7 Kishi S, Tso MOM, Hayreh SS: Fundus lesions in malignant hypertension. I. A pathologic study of experimental hypertensive choroidopathy. Arch Ophthalmol 1985;103:1189–1197.
8 Kishi S, Tso MOM, Hayreh SS: Fundus lesions in malignant hypertension. II. A pathologic study of experimental hypertensive optic neuropathy. Arch Ophthalmol 1985;103:1198–1206.
9 Hayreh SS, Servais GE, Virdi PS, et al: Fundus lesions in malignant hypertension. III. Arterial

blood pressure, biochemical and fundus changes. Ophthalmology 1986;93:45–59.
10 Hayreh SS, Servais GE, Virdi PS: Fundus lesions in malignant hypertension. IV. Focal intra-retinal periarteriolar transudates. Ophthalmology 1986;93:60–73.
11 Hayreh SS, Servais GE, Virdi PS: Fundus lesions in malignant hypertension. V. Hypertensive optic neuropathy. Ophthalmology 1986;93:74–87.
12 Hayreh SS, Servais GE, Virdi PS: Fundus lesions in malignant hypertension. VI. Hypertensive choroidopathy. Ophthalmology 1986;93:1383–1400.
13 Duke-Elder S, Dobree JH: System of Ophthalmology. Diseases of the Retina. London, Kimpton, 1967, vol 10, pp 141,330.
14 Ballantyne AJ, Michaelson IC: Textbook of the Fundus of the Eye. Edinburgh, Livingstone, 1970, p 179.
15 Wise GN, Dollery CT, Henkind P: The retinal circulation. New York, Harper & Row, 1971, p 331.
16 Dollery CT: Hypertensive retinopathy; in Genest J, Kuchel O, Hamet P, Cantin M (eds): Hypertension: Physiopathology and Treatment, ed 2. New York, McGraw-Hill, 1983, pp 723–832.
17 Hayreh SS, Servais GE, Virdi PS: Cotton-wool spots (inner retinal ischemic spots) in malignant arterial hypertension. Ophthalmologica 1989;198:197–215.
18 Hayreh SS, Servais GE, Virdi PS: Retinal arteriolar changes in malignant arterial hypertension. Ophthalmologica 1989;198:178–196.
19 Hayreh SS, Servais GE: Retinal hemorrhages in malignant arterial hypertension. Int Ophthalmol 1988;12:137–145, 197.
20 McGregor E, Isles CG, Jay JL, et al: Retinal changes in malignant hypertension. Br Med J 1986;292:233–234.
21 Michaelson IC, Eliakim M, Avshalom A, et al: An approach to the investigation of the vascular changes in the fundus of the eye in hypertension and arteriosclerosis; in Weigelin E (ed): Acta XX Conc Ophthalm Germania, part 1. Amsterdam, Excerpta Medica Foundation, 1967, pp 207–219.
22 Stokoe NL, Turner RWD: Normal retinal vascular patterns. Arterio-venous ratio as measure of arterial calibre. Br J Ophthalmol 1966;50:21–40.
23 Evelyn KA, Nicholls JVV, Turnbull W: A method of grading and recording. The retinal changes in essential hypertension. Am J Ophthalmol 1958;45:165–179.
24 Pickering GW: High Blood Pressure, ed 2. London, Churchill, 1968, p 449.

Dr. S. S. Hayreh
Department of Ophthalmology
University of Iowa Hospitals and Clinics
Iowa City, IA 52242 (USA)

Author Index

Subject Index

Ophthalmologica

Vol. 198, 1989

International Journal of Ophthalmology
Journal International d'Ophtalmologie
Internationale Zeitschrift für Augenheilkunde

Organ of the Netherlands Ophthalmological Society

Founded 1899 as 'Zeitschrift für Augenheilkunde'
by H. Kuhnt and J. von Michel
Continued by J. Meller (1923–1938), C. Behr (1925–1938),
A. Brückner (1938–1959), H.J.M. Weve (1938–1962),
H.M. Dekking (1954–1966), J. ten Doesschate (1967–1971),
J. François (1959–1979), E.B. Streiff (1954–1979), H. Sautter (1979–1984)

KARGER

Contents Vol. 198, 1989

S. Karger · Medical and Scientific Publishers
Basel · München · Paris · London · NewYork · New Delhi · Singapore · Tokyo · Sydney

Drug Dosage

The authors and the publisher have exerted every effort to ensure that drug selection and dosage set forth in this text are in accord with current recommendations and practice at the time of publication. However, in view of ongoing research, changes in government regulations, and the constant flow of information relating to drug therapy and drug reactions, the reader is urged to check the package insert for each drug for any change in indications and dosage and for added warnings and precautions. This is particularly important when the recommended agent is a new and/or infrequently employed drug.

Printed in Switzerland by
Buchdruckerei Friedrich Reinhardt AG, Basel